GREAT FEET *for* LIFE

Great Feet *for* Life

Footcare and Footwear
for Healthy Aging

PAUL LANGER, DPM

Fairview Press
Minneapolis

Published by Fairview Press, 2450 Riverside Avenue, Minneapolis, MN 55454. Fairview Press is a division of Fairview Health Services, a community-focused health system, affiliated with the University of Minnesota, providing a complete range of services, from the prevention of illness and injury to care for the most complex medical conditions.

For a free current catalog of Fairview Press titles, call toll-free 1-800-544-8207, or visit our Web site at www.fairviewpress.org.

Library of Congress Cataloging-in-Publication Data
Langer, Paul, 1966-
    Great feet for life : footcare and footwear for healthy aging / Paul Langer.
        p. cm.
    ISBN-13: 978-1-57749-159-0 (pbk. : alk. paper)
    ISBN-10: 1-57749-159-9 (pbk. : alk. paper)
    1. Foot—Care and hygiene. 2.   Footwear—Health aspects.   I. Title.
    RD563.L33 2007
    617.5'85--dc22

                                                                2006026941

Printed in the United States of America
First printing: March 2007
11 10 09 08 07   5 4 3 2 1

Cover by Laurie Ingram

Acknowledgments:
The author would like to express his appreciation to the following people for their assistance and expertise in preparing this book: Lane Stiles, Tim Larson, Steve Deger, Linda Lofgren, Jill Heaberlin, Sharon Healy, Kris Felsman, Jennifer Gundale, Michelle Corbo Langer, Robert Langer, Richard Corbo, and David Koehser.

For my parents, Patricia and Robert,
whose love and support made the fear of failure less daunting.

For my wife Michelle,
who has inspired me ever since that day I first saw her smile.

Contents

1

Appreciate Your Feet

According to the American Podiatric Medical Association, by age fifty the average person has walked 75,000 miles, or the equivalent of three laps around the earth. Though the human feet are marvelous shock absorbers, all these miles, ultimately, take a toll. After age thirty the human body begins to lose nerve function, muscle mass, bone mass, and flexibility. In addition, the fat pad on the bottom of the feet may start to atrophy, or shrink, resulting in less cushioning around the bones of the feet. And for many, the toes may start to curl as well. It has been well documented that foot problems increase with age. A European study found less the 3 percent of those over sixty had "normal" feet.[1]

To lead an active lifestyle it helps to have healthy feet. Healthy feet allow you to do many things that preserve your health and independence. Many of the most common chronic diseases are better managed by maintaining an active lifestyle. The damaging effects of heart disease, diabetes, circulation disorders, depression, obesity, and arthritis can be lessened by remaining active. Conversely, foot problems can compromise your health and independence. Losing the ability to walk, for example, leads to decreased self-esteem, social isolation, and a lower quality of life.[2] Even such simple activities as grocery shopping or gardening can become difficult, if not impossible, without the firm foundation provided by healthy feet.

As important as they are for good health, the feet may be the most neglected part of the human body. Because painful conditions of the feet are so common, many people assume that foot pain is just a normal part of everyday life and that there is nothing they can do about it. Sometimes medical professionals can become so busy managing other medical conditions that the feet get little attention. If we all appreciated our feet a bit more, we might take better care of them.

Consider this: With each step you take, your body lands with one to one and a half times your weight. Since most of us take between five and ten thousand steps a day, the total impact on our feet quickly adds up. In fact, the average 150-pound person absorbs as much as 1.5 million pounds of step impact through his or her feet each day. Over the course of a year, this would add up to more than 400 million pounds of total weight. For a 225-pound person, the annual impact could easily exceed 600 million pounds!

Fortunately, these high impact forces can be absorbed very efficiently by healthy feet and legs. The skin, muscles, bones, and connective tissue of the feet and legs are amazingly strong and resilient—*if* well cared for. However, there are three forces conspiring against the feet to cause us all misery and pain:

(1) *We begin to wear shoes at too early an age.*

In developed countries, we begin putting shoes on children before they can even walk. Human feet are designed to bear weight on natural surfaces without restriction from footwear. When confined by shoes, the muscles that support the arch and maintain alignment of the toes are not able to develop properly. The developing feet of a child do not need artificial support or cushioning. These things actually hinder the development of foot strength and flexibility by preventing or delaying normal muscular and neurological development.

One study has found that barefoot toddlers learn to walk sooner and fall less than those wearing shoes.[3] As we age, the muscular development that we missed out on as children causes imbalances in our feet that can lead to painful conditions, including hammer toes and heel pain. Most of these painful conditions take decades to manifest and may not even be noticeable until age thirty or later.

(2) We tend to wear shoes that don't fit us properly.

Some types of shoes are obviously not good for our feet: shoes that squeeze our feet into unnatural shapes or cramped spaces—high heels or cowboy boots, for example. But even some athletic shoes can be surprisingly bad for our feet as well. Shoe fashions and shoe cushioning are quietly changing the alignment of our joints and weakening the muscles of our feet with each of the five to ten thousand steps we take daily. In the name of fashion, many people overlook the possibility that long-term use of unhealthy shoes can cause significant foot deformities and pain later in life. And while many people assume that cushioning is the answer to all types of foot pain, too much cushioning in footwear can destabilize the feet so much that impact forces actually increase during walking.

(3) We walk on unnaturally hard surfaces.

Artificial surfaces such as concrete and asphalt are everywhere, but human feet were not intended to stand on concrete, which is fifty times harder than the earth. Hard surfaces have been linked to arthritis and back pain. Concrete is hiding under the carpet at work, at the library, at the mall, and in hospitals. Even the tile floors in homes can be too hard for the healthy function of feet.

In developed countries, unnaturally hard surfaces can be hard to avoid. Work, home, stores, airports, even health clubs and restaurants often have walking surfaces that are dramatically harder than natural surfaces. Carpet or rubber mats cannot always compensate for the increased strain that these surfaces place on the human body.

Keep in mind that while going barefoot, walking on natural surfaces, and wearing properly fitting shoes does not guarantee that the feet will be healthier in later years, research has shown that shoe-wearing populations do have a high incidence of foot problems. Problems with the feet can limit mobility and decrease quality of life. Fortunately, most foot problems can be easily addressed. Before we consider the various problems that can affect the feet, though, it might help to take a quick look at foot anatomy and physiology. This may help us better appreciate how the feet can be both resilient and injury-prone at the same time.

Most Common Foot Complaints by Older Adults

	toenail problems	skin problems	calluses or corns	swelling	bunions	arthritis
women	29%	29%	27%	25%	25%	22%
men	28%	11%	12%	10%	8%	23%

Source: Munro, BJ, Steele, JR, "Footcare awareness: a survey of persons aged 65 and older," *Journal of the American Podiatric Medical Association*, 88 (5): 242–248, 1988.

Foot structure

The foot is made up of 28 bones. In fact, one-fourth of all the bones in the human skeleton are located within the feet. The bones of the feet are small compared to the bones of the other weight-bearing parts of the body. Although sharing remarkable similarities with the bones of the hand, foot bones have adapted to weight-bearing stress by becoming denser and stronger than the corresponding bones of the hands. In effect, the small foot bones make up in strength what they lack in size. Bone is capable of responding to the stress placed on it. For example, heavier people have denser bones than lighter people, and runners have denser bones than swimmers.

The small bones of the foot, and the soft tissue structures that connect them, are arranged in a way that enable the foot to create an arch that can collapse and spring back as weight is transferred from the heels to the toes during each step. The structures of the foot are specialized to withstand the demands of weight-bearing activity. For example, the skin on the bottom of the foot is twice as thick as skin on the rest of the body and contains millions of specialized nerve fibers that help us to maintain our balance. Tendons, which connect the muscles to the bones, transmit to the foot the tremendous forces that are generated by the large muscles of the hip and leg. Ligaments, which connect the bones to one another, help keep the joints aligned. Blood flow supplies the oxygen to the cells of the foot, and fat provides cushioning to the bottom of the foot.

The complexity of the foot's structure allows it to perform difficult work over long periods of time. But this complexity can also contribute to a potential for injury and other problems. More than 100 joints, tendons, muscles, and ligaments hold the elaborate architecture of the foot together. Over time, the cartilage that cushions the joints from impact and reduces friction between the bones can wear down, resulting in arthritis. The joint at the base of the big toe can be affected by bunions or gout. Painful flat feet can result when joints become unstable. Overuse can cause tendons to become inflamed. Overstretching can damage ligaments, causing inflammation, sprains, and even dislocated joints.

The nerves make up another complex system in the feet. More than simply transmitting sensations and stimulating muscle contractions, the nerves in the feet help regulate temperature and blood flow, hydrate the skin, and, very importantly, maintain balance. The loss of nerve function in the feet greatly contributes to the risk of falling.

There is also a complex circulatory system in the feet. Arteries bring oxygenated blood to the feet, and veins bring oxygen-depleted blood back to the heart. Gravity forces this circulatory system to work hard to return blood all the way from the feet up to the heart. This is why the feet can be susceptible to swelling. Because the working muscles of the legs and feet demand more oxygen during walking and running than the muscles in the upper body, poor blood flow can cause pain and fatigue in these muscles. Heart disease, high blood pressure, and other disorders can also cause pain and swelling in the feet and legs.

You may not think of fat as a type of foot structure, but a special type of fat is instrumental in helping to cushion the foot from the impact of walking and running. The plantar fat pad is a dense layer of fat on the bottom of the foot that is especially thick under the heel. Even though many of us find ourselves gaining unwanted fat as we age, plantar fat may actually start to shrink with age. A shrinking fat pad makes it more difficult to soften impact and can cause bones to protrude on the bottom or sides of the foot, making it vulnerable to pressure-related pain.

Biomechanics

The term *biomechanics* refers to how the living structures of the human body move. How well our muscles, joints, bones, and tendons work together determines how efficiently our body moves. Clearly, the complexity of the foot's structure means that its biomechanics are also very complex. The feet have to be flexible enough to absorb repeated impact and adapt to variable walking surfaces but rigid enough to support the weight of the body and propel it forward.

As it turns out, the feet have an amazing ability to alternate between being a "flexible adapter" and a "rigid lever." The major joints of the foot working together are capable of two distinct motions referred to as "pronation" and "supination." When we take a step, certain joints of the foot unlock, allowing it to flex in order to absorb impact. This is pronation. It occurs just after the heel strikes the ground and continues as the weight of the body is transferred to the front, or ball, of the foot. As the heel then starts to lift from the ground, the joints lock again to become a rigid lever pushing the body forward. This is supination. These motions occur in tenths of seconds when walking and mere hundredths of seconds when running.

The complexity of these movements increases the potential for biomechanical problems to develop. If your feet are too flexible and unstable, we say that you have "overpronation." Overpronation strains the bones and soft tissues of the feet and lower legs and can even strain the knees, hips, and lower back in severe cases. If your feet are too rigid, we say that you have "oversupination." Oversupination can lead to ankle sprains and impact-induced injuries. Overpronation is much more common than oversupination. In general, those with flat feet are the most severe overpronators, while those with extremely high arches are the most severe oversupinators.

At least once a week a patient will come to my clinic and proclaim that their arches have "fallen." While it is not unusual for the feet to change shape and size as we age, it is unusual for arches to fall. A condition called posterior tibial tendon dysfunction can lead to a flattening of the arch, but this condition is uncommon, typically affecting those who already have flat feet.

Foot types

While it is an oversimplification to say that all feet fall into one of three basic types, it is sometimes useful to think about feet in this way—for instance, when buying shoes or treating minor foot injuries. Each foot type has its own special characteristics and its own vulnerability to certain kinds of injuries. The three basic foot types, based on the height of the arches, are

- high
- normal or neutral
- low or flat.

High

People with high arches may have a history of repeated or severe ankle sprains. High arches tend to make the feet more rigid and less efficient at absorbing step impact. High arches also make it less likely that shoes can provide support, so flexible and cushioned footwear is usually more comfortable than stiff or firm footwear.

Normal or neutral

As mentioned above, normal arches fall somewhere between low and high arches. This is, of course, a subjective judgment. People with neutral arches tend to be the most efficient at absorbing impact and transferring weight from heel to toes during walking and running, though they can be vulnerable to some of the same injuries that those with low arches experience. A neutral foot is more versatile in terms of what kinds of shoes or insoles are comfortable.

Low or flat

People with low arches may have a history of arch pain, tendonitis, and, in severe cases, arthritis of the feet or knees. Yet some people with low arches have no foot problems at all. Flat feet are a severe form of low arches and are best evaluated and treated by a podiatrist or orthopedist. Symptoms of flat feet can be made worse by wearing shoes that lack support.

Determining Foot Type

While a podiatrist or orthopedic doctor can more accurately assess your foot, there is a simple self-test you can do to get a general idea of your foot type. Simply wet your foot and step onto a paper towel. When you step off, a high arch will leave a curved shape in the area between the toes and heel. A low or flat arch will fill in the area under the arch between the toes and heel. A normal or neutral arch will fall somewhere in between. Keep in mind that approximately 80 percent of the population will be somewhere in the normal range of arch height based on this self-assessment. Only the flattest arches or highest arches are easily identifiable, and each accounts for only 10 percent of the general population. Having an extremely high or extremely low arch does not necessarily doom you to injury, nor does having a normal or neutral foot type make you immune to injury.

A complete and accurate biomechanical foot exam can only be done by a medical practitioner. The exam involves not only the determination of foot type but also an assessment of range of motion, walking gait, shoe wear patterns, and X-rays of the foot while standing. A complete exam is not limited to the feet. The doctor will examine arm swing, the alignment of the shoulder and head, the movement of the hips and pelvis, and leg function to gather a complete picture of how the feet support and coordinate the movement of the body.

Foot width

One final aspect of the physiology of feet is worth mentioning here: foot width. Foot width is sometimes more of a concern for women than men for two reasons:

(1) Our culture expects women to have petite feet.

(2) Manufacturers do not offer many shoes for women in wide sizes (though even men may have limited choices if they have especially wide feet).

There are many different types of wide feet. Some feet are wide from heel to toe; some are narrow in the heel and wide in the forefoot. Bunions or arthritis can cause our feet to widen very gradually. Aging can also cause our feet to widen. While there is no specific clinical definition for wide feet, we know that wider feet are more vulnerable to certain types of injuries, including neuromas, corns, and toe calluses. For more information on foot width, see the chapter on shoes later in this book.

Appreciating the anatomy and physiology of our feet is the first step toward understanding how to care for and treat our feet. The following chapters will discuss specific foot conditions and how to treat them.

Footcare Specialists

Podiatrists and **orthopedists** are doctors who diagnose and treat foot injuries and diseases.

Podiatrists specialize in medical care of the foot, ankle, and lower leg. A podiatrist must have a doctor of podiatric medicine (DPM) degree.

Orthopedists (also spelled **orthopaedists**) specialize in problems relating to bones, joints, and muscles. Orthopedists treat problems throughout the body, not just the feet.

After a diagnosis has been made, **certified pedorthists**, **pharmacists**, **footcare nurses**, and **physical therapists** may be involved in treatment.

Pedorthists should not be confused with podiatrists. Pedorthists use foot devices and footwear to help relieve foot problems. A **certified pedorthist** (C.Ped.) is a pedorthist who has gone through special training and certification.

Knowledgeable shoe store employees can advise you about appropriate footwear and help fit you properly. But be careful. Shoe store employees who are not properly trained can provide poor advice. Shoe store employees are not qualified to diagnose or treat medical conditions or injuries. In fact, a well-trained retail employee will make a point of stating this if questioned about a foot problem.

Recently, retail foot-comfort centers have become more common. Retail chains such as Foot Solutions and Eneslow Foot Comfort Centers often employ or are owned by certified pedorthists. Foot-comfort centers offer foot devices and footwear designed to maximize foot comfort and foot health.

2

Skin Care

The skin is the largest organ of the body and our main barrier to infection. It is often said that our skin is a window to our overall health. It can indicate how well we're eating, exercising, and taking care of ourselves. It also can reveal signs of chronic diseases, such as diabetes, rheumatoid arthritis, thyroid disorders, and heart disease. Even the effects of long-term smoking can be seen in the quality of our skin.

Taking care of the skin of the feet is extremely important to good foot health. The demands on the skin of the feet are unique because of the extraordinary amount of wear and tear the feet must bear. Not only must the skin of the feet be strong enough to withstand the continuous pounding of walking and running, but it must also be elastic enough to stretch as the feet bend and move. The skin on the bottom of the feet is twice as thick as the skin on any other part of the body and has a dense pad of fat underneath it (called the plantar fat pad) to cushion and protect the bones of the feet. Any compromise to the integrity of the skin of the feet, such as a calluses, corns, blisters, or cracking, can cause pain, infections, and even injury.

Though not common, moles, "freckles," or "old age spots" can sometimes be cancerous. Suspicious moles on the feet should be evaluated by your doctor. A painless mole that has been present for years without any obvious changes should be measured and documented by your doctor so that it can be monitored on a regular basis. Newly discovered moles or moles that have changed in size or color should be monitored as well.

Changes in our skin as we age

As we age, the appearance and texture of our skin change. Blood flow decreases, which causes the skin to become drier, thinner, and less elastic. The color of the skin changes as well, and less hair grows on the lower legs and feet. The glands in our skin produce less sweat and oil. In addition, the plantar fat pad can shrink, resulting in less cushioning around the bones. This can cause painful calluses to form on the forefoot and toes. A study in Spain found that 78 percent of study subjects age sixty and older had skin conditions of the feet, with calluses being the most common finding. This study also found that more than 70 percent of the subjects had both skin conditions and other foot disorders, such as bunions, toenail changes, and contracted toes. Fewer than 3 percent had "normal" feet.[4]

Some of us experience numbness or lack of feeling in our feet as we age due to a loss of nerve function called peripheral neuropathy. Loss of nerve function can make it more difficult to detect other problems with our feet, such as calluses or blisters. Over time, this can lead to much more serious problems, including open sores and infection. Changes in the nerves as we age can also make our feet more sensitive to burning sensations and less able to regulate the temperature of our skin.

Numbness and peripheral neuropathy will be discussed in more detail in the chapter on nerve conditions. For now, however, a word of caution: If you have numbness or lack of feeling in your feet, you should be extremely careful with your skin and inspect your feet daily. Do not attempt to care for your skin and toenails by yourself. Instead, seek the advice and care of a doctor—if possible, a podiatrist.

Because of changes in our skin as we age, our feet and lower legs can become vulnerable to certain skin conditions and less resistant to calluses, infections, and even ulcers. Thin skin tears easily and heals slowly. This chapter will discuss some of the more common skin conditions of the feet and offer suggestions on how to care for them. Basic skin hygiene and callus care are things we can do for ourselves. More serious skin problems, such as painful skin conditions, rashes, or infections, should be treated by a podiatrist, dermatologist, or general practitioner.

Skin hygiene

Foot hygiene can become increasingly difficult as we age. For example, poor vision, arthritic hands, and poor balance can make it difficult to care for or even reach the feet. Simple tasks such as applying lotion, bathing the feet, and especially trimming the toenails can be extremely difficult tasks. Those who cannot see or reach their feet must rely on family members or caregivers to assist with daily foot hygiene.

A European study suggested that poor foot hygiene was the first event in a gradual decline in foot health that ultimately leads to foot pain and limited mobility.[5] Accumulating dirt, moisture, fungus, and bacteria contribute to odors and infections of the skin and discoloration and thickening of the toenails. Poor foot hygiene can also be a source of embarrassment for some, with a surprisingly negative effect on self-image.[6] Fortunately, good foot hygiene is a very effective way to maintain health and prevent foot problems.

Washing the skin on a daily basis is the first step in keeping the feet healthy. In addition, clean, comfortable socks and breathable shoes help to decrease the risk of fungal injections (e.g., athlete's foot), bacterial and viral infections between the toes, and foot odor. Proper cleaning of the feet involves

- washing with soap and water;
- drying the skin thoroughly;
- using powders, lotions, or topical antifungal medications as needed.

Moisturize dry skin with lotions, and treat dry, moist, or sweaty skin with powders. Treating athlete's foot or other fungal infections diligently with topical antifungals is especially important to minimize the risk of fungal nails. Finally, good foot hygiene requires good shoe and sock care. Old shoes and unwashed socks can harbor bacteria and fungus. Wear a fresh pair of socks each day and replace old, smelly, worn-out shoes. If you use a communal shower, such as at a health club, wear shower sandals to protect your feet against the funguses and bacteria that flourish on locker room floors.

Problems affecting the skin of the feet

On the following pages are some common problems affecting the skin of the feet and some general advice about how to address these problems. Remember that this advice is for information only and is not meant to replace the advice of your doctor or other health care professionals.

The skin problems discussed in this chapter include:

- dry skin
- moist skin between the toes
- sweaty or smelly feet
- athlete's foot
- blisters
- itching skin, including eczema, psoriasis, allergic reactions, and parasitic infestations
- bacterial infections
- skin changes associated with blood flow, including purpura, venous stasis dermatitis, hemosiderin deposits, Raynaud's disease/phenomenon, and fragile or "thin" skin
- plantar warts
- calluses and corns, including underlying injuries, cracking skin, pressure ulcers, and seed corns (porokeratosis).

Dry skin

Dry skin can result from poor nutrition, dehydration, decreased blood flow, weather changes, smoking, or simply a normal part of the aging process. Our skin produces less oil as we age, which naturally results in drier skin. There are a number of infections and diseases that can cause dry skin as well. Athlete's foot is a common cause of dry skin and is discussed later in this chapter. Soap can also dry our skin. Some soaps are harsher than others, so consider switching to a milder soap if dryness is a persistent problem.

Basic dry skin without redness, cracking, blistering, scaling, or open sores can usually be treated with moisturizing lotion or cream. Applied once daily—or, in drier climates, twice daily—most moisturizing lotions work quite well.

For persistent dry skin that flakes or develops into a thick callus, moisturizing creams or lotions that also have a gentle exfoliating acid may be helpful. Ingredients such as alpha hydroxyl acids (glycolic or lactic acid) or urea can help to dissolve the dry skin while moisturizing the healthy skin. Creams are thicker and work better on extremely dry skin but can feel greasy. Lotions are better for daily use and feel less greasy. Eucerin, Kerasal, AmLactin or Carmol are brands of lotions and creams that work effectively. But since they come in a number of varieties, make sure that the product you select contains an exfoliating agent. Product labels that use such terms as "for extra dry skin" or "for tough, scaly skin" usually contain one or more exfoliating agents. Be aware, though, that these ingredients can irritate the skin if used too often or if used on skin that is not dry and scaling. They can also make the skin more sensitive to the effects of the sun. Some people find that they only need the exfoliating lotion during the winter months or periodically when dry skin builds up.

The best time to apply moisturizing lotion is immediately after gently toweling dry following a bath or shower. Application of lotion after bathing helps to retain the moisture of the shower or bath water on your skin.

Unless directed to by your doctor, moisturizing lotions or creams should never be applied between the toes. The skin there can become excessively moist with lotions. This excessive moisture can provide a breeding ground for bacteria and fungus. Dry skin between the toes is most often a sign of athlete's foot or other skin condition and should be treated with medication rather than a moisturizer.

Moist skin between the toes

Excessive moisture between the toes can cause the skin to break down, or "macerate." Macerated skin appears white and sloughs off as it weakens and breaks down. Macerated skin is vulnerable to fungal and bacterial infections, which can cause redness, itching, and cracking. If your feet perspire excessively and are vulnerable to repeated athlete's foot infections, you are

Weave a thin strip of lamb's wool between your toes to help alleviate excessive moisture.

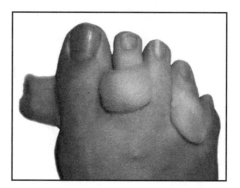

more likely to have maceration between your toes. To treat excessive moisture between your toes, carefully dry your skin after bathing, apply foot powder, and weave a thin strip of lamb's wool between your toes. Allowing the feet to "air out" also helps. For stubborn cases, antifungals, antibiotics, or drying agents may be prescribed by a podiatrist.

Sweaty or smelly feet

Hyperhidrosis is a condition where the sweat glands of the feet and hands are overactive, resulting in excessive sweating. Many things, including stress, changes in the weather, illness, and medications, can trigger an episode of excessive sweating. Most often, we don't know what the trigger is.

Excessive moisture on the skin can lead to such problems as foot odor, athlete's foot, blisters, and warts. The bad odor we associate with sweaty feet is usually caused by bacteria or fungi that thrive in the warm, moist confines of shoes. And while moisture does not itself cause blisters or warts, it can weaken the skin making it more susceptible to blisters and warts.

Unfortunately, there is no cure for hyperhidrosis. Most treatments are aimed at keeping the feet dry. First and foremost, it is important that sufferers wear shoes made from "breathable" materials (materials that allow air to move into and out of the shoe). For casual or dress shoes, leather uppers tend to be more breathable than synthetic leather. Nylon mesh uppers are ideal, especially for sporting activities.

Socks are important for preventing and treating hyperhidrosis because they can either trap moisture next to the skin or help it to evaporate. Contrary to popular belief, cotton is not the ideal fabric for socks, because when cotton gets wet, it stays wet. Though soft and absorbent, cotton is not as effective as newer fabrics at protecting the skin of the feet. Nylon and other synthetic materials can wick, or pull, moisture away from the skin and help it to evaporate. All shoe stores and sporting goods stores carry socks that wick moisture from the skin. But wicking socks have their limitations, so even these socks should be changed two or more times a day if the feet are particularly sweaty.

Topical skin treatments can also help control excessive moisture.

Powders are very effective at keeping the feet cool and dry. Most powders are made from talc or cornstarch, or a combination of the two. For those with sensitive skin, cornstarch-based powders may be less irritating. Foot powders that include an antifungal ingredient are especially useful for those with athlete's foot. It is best to apply the powder directly to the feet instead of sprinkling it into the socks or shoes.

Powdering the skin directly is more effective than putting powder in the shoes or socks. A simple way to powder the feet is to cover the bottom of a small pan or shoe box with powder and dip the feet in before putting on socks and shoes.

Some roll-on and powder products contain the antiperspirant aluminum chloride and can decrease sweating when applied daily. They also work well in combination with the other treatments described in this section. Aluminum chloride products are available without prescription at many stores and pharmacies.

Soaking the feet in a solution of one part aluminum acetate diluted in twenty parts water (called Burrow's solution), followed by an application of an exfoliating lotion, can help in some cases. The addition of foot soaking to a regimen of daily use of powders can work well for stubborn cases of foot odor and sweating feet.

Athlete's foot

Athlete's foot is an infection of the skin caused by a fungus. Fungus is always living on our skin. Most of the time, this fungus is held in check by our immune system. Occasionally, however, when conditions are right, the fungus can overwhelm our natural defenses and flare up, by either rapidly reproducing on the surface of the skin or by infecting tiny scrapes or tears in the skin.

Free your feet from your shoes whenever possible to let them "breathe." The dark, moist, warm environment created by shoes is a breeding ground for bacteria and fungus. Sandals are great for warm climates and seasons, and for those whose feet sweat heavily or are prone to odor. In colder climates and during colder seasons, changing socks frequently helps keep the feet dry.

Fungus thrives on warm, moist surfaces, such as the insides of shoes and shower floors. Everyone is susceptible to athlete's foot, but outbreaks are most common in people whose feet sweat profusely, especially during warm months. Just as some of us are more susceptible than others to colds or allergies, some of us are more susceptible to fungal infections. Often, susceptibility is a family trait.

Do not treat a suspected case of athlete's foot with anything other than an antifungal medication unless directed to do so by a doctor. Topical cortisone creams can actually make the infection worse, and topical antibiotics can promote growth of resistant forms of bacteria.

The most common symptoms of athlete's foot are redness with itching, flaking skin on the bottoms of the feet. Some forms of athlete's foot cause moist, white, peeling skin between the toes or small fluid-filled blisters on the arch. Other symptoms include burning and odor. If untreated, athlete's foot can contribute to fungal infection of the toenails and secondary bacterial skin infections. Even with diligent treatment some people are vulnerable to recurrences.

Treatment of athlete's foot involves good foot hygiene, topical medications, and frequent shoe and sock changes. Foot hygiene requires bathing the feet daily in soap and water and drying them thoroughly, especially in between the toes. Keeping the skin dry by using foot powders and wearing ventilated shoes is also important. Old, smelly shoes should be thrown away to prevent reinfection. Suffers should wear clean socks every day. Clean socks help keep the feet dry and, most important, minimize the amount of fungus on the skin. For those whose feet tend to sweat profusely, changing socks two or three times a day is beneficial.

In addition to good foot hygiene, treatment of athlete's foot requires medication. Seventy to 80 percent of athlete's foot infections respond to topical, over-the-counter treatments. A doctor's care may be needed for stubborn cases of athlete's foot (those that do not respond to treatment within one to two weeks). He or she may run diagnostic lab tests to confirm the diagnosis and to decide if treatment with prescription medication is necessary.

Sloughing, or peeling, skin between the toes can be a sign of a particularly stubborn form of athlete's foot that involves a bacterial infection as well as the fungal infection. This form is most commonly seen between the fourth and fifth toes. Treatment is the

Treat athlete's foot for one to two weeks after the symptoms have disappeared and use an antifungal powder daily thereafter to minimize the risk of recurrence.

same as that for other athlete's foot outbreaks: wash and thoroughly dry the feet and apply an antifungal powder on a daily basis. In some cases, placing swatches of cotton or lamb's wool between the toes is also helpful. Keeping the areas between the toes as dry as possible will promote healing. Sufferers should see a doctor if an outbreak does not respond within two weeks. A prescription medication may be required.

Blisters

Blisters on the feet can be caused by drug reactions, infections, allergic reactions, or friction (rubbing)—most commonly, the friction created by wearing new shoes. In severe cases, blood will fill the blisters and cause them to appear purple or black. Shoes that are too wide usually cause blisters in the arch or the bottom of the forefoot. Shoes that do not have enough toe length or toe depth will cause blisters on the tops or sides of the toes. Shoes that are too stiff or too loose in the heel will cause blisters on the back of the heels.

Always break in new shoes gradually, making sure to remove them at the first sign of pain. (More information on how to break in new shoes can be found in the shoe chapter.)

The safest way to treat a friction blister is to remove the shoe, cover the blister with a bandage (bandages especially made for blisters are now available at most pharmacies), and monitor the site for signs of infection. If you have a circulation disorder, thin skin, or diabetes, you should be especially cautious with blisters. Do not stick any adhesive bandages directly to the blister itself, as this could tear the skin on removal. Adhesive bandages should only stick to the healthy skin around the blister.

Once a blister has broken open or drained, it should be treated as any open sore and monitored for signs of infection. Treat the site with a topical antibiotic and cover with a bandage. If the blister is painful and does not drain or break open, it should be seen by a doctor. Likewise, see a doctor if a blister shows signs of infection (growing redness around the site, presence of pus). To avoid infection, it is best to have a medical professional drain the fluid from the blister. A doctor can also best diagnose and treat a blister that is infected.

If a medical professional is not readily available and the blister is in a place that limits walking ability, you may drain it carefully yourself. Keep in mind that a blister that is punctured or breaks open is much more likely to become infected than a blister that remains intact. Blisters that are red or purple in color likely contain blood and should not be punctured. Ideally, you should clean the skin around the blister with iodine or similar antiseptic before attempting to drain it. At the very least, scrub the area vigorously with soap and water. You can sterilize a sewing needle or safety pin by either boiling it in water for fifteen minutes or holding it to a flame and then cleaning it with isopropyl alcohol. The blister can then be pierced at its lowest point so that gravity will help it drain. Rolling a finger over the blister toward the hole where you pierced it will help to squeeze out the fluid. Occasionally the blister will require two to three punctures to drain. Drain all of the fluid to alleviate the discomfort the blister is causing you, but do not remove the skin of the blister. Protect, cover, and monitor the site of the blister for signs of infection. Eventually, the blistered skin will dry up and slough off as it heals.

Blisters that are the result of a drug reaction, infection, or allergic reaction usually appear as clusters of blisters with red skin surrounding them. These should be covered with a bandage and seen by a medical professional as soon as possible, as they could be a sign of a serious medical condition.

Itching skin

Itching skin is very common. It can be caused by a number of things, including certain medications, changes in blood flow, infections, parasites, allergic reactions, and skin conditions (such as eczema and psoriasis). Most commonly, itching skin of the feet is caused by athlete's foot or, simply, dryness.

Itching feet can be treated by moisturizing the skin with lotion. For stubborn cases, you can apply a nonprescription antihistamine or cortisone cream in addition to the moisturizer. Be careful, however, not to treat athlete's foot with cortisone cream because this could make the condition worse. Contact your doctor if itching persists.

Some skin changes are more difficult to diagnose and treat. The conditions listed below should be evaluated by a medical professional so that appropriate treatment can be initiated.

Eczema

Eczema is condition where dry, scaly, itchy patches of skin form on the lower legs or feet. Outbreaks are sometimes also found on the trunk or arms as well. There are a few different forms of eczema, each with its own unique characteristics. The skin lesions may be caused by allergic reactions, nutritional deficiencies, hereditary factors, or circulation changes. The dry, itching skin can crack, bleed, or break open if it is scratched. Emoliants, topical cortisone cream, and petroleum jelly are often used to treat eczema. Occasionally, however, topical or oral antibiotics are needed if a secondary infection develops. Treatment is dependent on which type of eczema is present. For this reason, you should see a doctor if you think you have eczema.

Psoriasis

Psoriasis is a hereditary skin disorder that causes skin lesions, swelling, and arthritis. It appears as itchy patches of silvery scales on the elbows, scalp, forearms, back, hands, or feet. It can make wearing shoes and socks uncomfortable and even painful. While 75 percent of those with psoriasis are affected at an early age, 25 percent do not see symptoms until age fifty or later.

Psoriasis of the feet is best evaluated and treated by a rheumatologist or a dermatologist working with a podiatrist. Without proper treatment, psoriasis is persistent and can even become infected. And, although it is not contagious, it can spread to affect larger patches of skin. To the untrained eye, psoriasis can be confused with calluses or athlete's foot and, therefore, may not be treated properly. Contact a doctor if you think you may have psoriasis.

Allergic reactions

Allergic reactions can cause itching, redness, hives, bumps, and blisters. The most common causes of allergic reactions on the skin of the feet are new shoes, new socks, new laundry detergent, or a bandage. In fact, a good indication of an allergic reaction is that often the irritated area has the shape of whatever caused the reaction, such as straps from a sandal. Leather is not usually an allergen, but shoe leather may contain other materials, such as synthetics, dyes, or adhesives, that do cause allergic reactions. Many socks contain synthetic elastic fibers that can cause or contribute to rashes. Latex and other synthetic rubbers are highly allergenic for some people.

In addition to what people put over their feet, what they put on their feet can also trigger or contribute to allergic reactions. Adhesives found in tapes or bandages are allergens for some. And some people are allergic to creams, lotions, powders, and even topical antibiotics. Of special concern are over-the-counter corn and callus treatments. In people with poor circulation, diabetes, or numbness, these treatments can cause severe skin reactions.

Sometimes allergens get on the skin unintentionally. People who are allergic to plants such as poison ivy and poison oak should wash off any oily residue with soap and water as quickly as possible in order to minimize the severity of the skin reaction.

Some allergic reactions are caused by what people put into the body. People who take multiple medications may be vulnerable to generalized skin rashes. If a change in or an addition of medications has preceded a rash outbreak, inform the prescribing physician immediately. Such a rash is a sign of a serious side effect and should be evaluated by a medical professional. Foods and drink can also cause allergic reactions. As with medications, suspected food and drink allergies should be immediately evaluated by a physician.

Basic treatment of an allergic reaction on the feet consists of washing the skin, applying a powder to absorb moisture and residual allergens, and using a topical cortisone cream to decrease the itching, inflammation, and redness. Of course, you should also remove the suspected triggering agent(s). If the itching and rash do not respond to treatment, consult a physician.

Parasitic infestations

Parasite infestations can be intensely itchy, especially at night. The parasite burrows under the skin leaving a curved track that can be seen in the itching area. Sometimes there are small blisters present as well. Norwegian or keratotic scabies can produce white scales under and around the toenails and then spread to the surrounding skin. Suspected parasite infestations should be diagnosed and treated by a physician.

Bacterial infections

Signs of bacterial infection of the skin include pain, redness, draining, swelling, and pitting and sloughing of the skin. In severe infections, malaise, loss of appetite, fever, chills, nausea, and vomiting can occur. It is always safest to have a suspected infection evaluated by a medical professional. Anyone experiencing symptoms of infection should seek immediate medical attention.

There are several common bacterial infections of the foot. Pitted keratolysis is a minor bacterial infection where small, dark pits typically form on the heels, though some people may have other symptoms. In some cases, these pitted lesions cause itching and discomfort. A doctor may prescribe an antibiotic medication if there is itching and discomfort.

An ingrown toenail can puncture the skin and cause a painful bacterial infection, commonly on the big toe. In minor cases, soaking the infected toe in warm soapy water twice daily and covering the site with iodine or a topical antibiotic and a bandage can help heal the infection. Check the nail and remove any sharp edges that may be the cause of the infection. For recurrent infections, a podiatrist may need to care for the nail. See the chapter on nails for more information.

Feet that sweat excessively are especially vulnerable to an infection that may mimic a bacterial infection but is caused by a type of fungus known as yeast. *Candida albicans* is a common yeast that thrives in warm, moist environments, which makes the skin between the toes an ideal location for infection. White, sloughing skin with surrounding redness is a sign of *Candida albicans* infection. This yeast infection is often mistaken for athlete's foot, but is not treatable with some of the more common over-the-counter athlete's foot medications. If a suspected case of athlete's foot does not improve after two to three days of using topical antifungal medications, then a bacterial or candida infection may be present. Seek care from a medical professional.

Skin changes associated with blood flow

If the flow of blood to the lower legs and feet changes, the color and texture of the skin may also change. Changes in blood flow can also increase the risk of certain types of skin conditions. In fact, many skin changes of the feet and lower legs can be the first signs of developing blood flow disorders. Below are a few of the more common conditions associated with changes in blood flow.

Purpura

Purpura (also called cherry angioma or senile angioma) is a rash of brownish-red, bright-red, or purple spots that may gradually change to brown over time. The small spots are actually sites of tiny, ruptured blood vessels. They can be caused by an allergic reaction, anemia, or a systemic condition such as vascular disease, but most often are simply a normal part of aging.

Venous stasis dermatitis

Venous stasis dermatitis is an inflammation of the skin that can occur with varicose veins or swelling in the lower legs or feet. The circulation of blood through affected areas is slowed, causing itching, redness, and brown patches. Shiny, thin, weakened skin may also result. This thin and weakened skin is vulnerable to tearing and heals slowly. In severe cases, the skin can break down, forming weeping, open sores called venous stasis ulcers. Treatments for venous stasis dermatitis include wearing compression stockings, periodically elevating the legs, exercising, and treating any sores that may be present.

Hemosiderin deposits

Hemosiderin deposits are painless brown patches of skin that form on the lower legs. They can occur when the legs swell, constricting and backing up the flow of blood. The backed-up blood flow deposits iron in the skin, causing the brown spots. Treatment is directed at controlling the swelling. The discolored skin, however, is harmless and often remains for years.

Raynaud's disease/phenomenon

Raynaud's disease/phenomenon is a vascular condition in which small blood vessels in the fingers and toes spasm, causing changes in temperature and color changes to the skin. The disease can also cause numbness and pain. In the most severe cases, Raynaud's disease/phenomenon can lead to gangrene.

The vascular spasms can be set off by stress or weather changes and can cause the skin to appear white, blue, or red, depending on what stage it is in. (Those who have experienced prolonged exposure to cold or frostbite are vulnerable to a similar condition called chilblain, or pernio.)

Raynaud's disease/phenomenon should be diagnosed by a physician. Keeping the skin warm is the primary treatment. Wearing warm socks and shoes and avoiding cold exposure to the feet often keeps symptoms in control. Prescription medications that increase blood flow may also be used to treat severe cases.

Fragile or "thin" skin

Peripheral vascular disease (also known as peripheral artery disease, or PAD), thyroid disorders, and long-term use of oral steroids can cause the skin to become thin and fragile. Affected skin often has a texture like rice paper and is easily injured. Even a slight bump can severely bruise or tear the skin. Bruises and the smallest tears can take weeks to heal. Those with fragile skin have to be extremely careful walking barefoot or breaking in new shoes and should visually inspect their feet and lower legs every day. Cuts or skin tears usually heal slowly and should be covered and checked regularly to ensure that they do not become infected.

Plantar warts

Plantar warts are found on the plantar surface (bottom) of the foot and are caused by a virus. They are often confused with calluses and are not properly treated. Even when correctly identified, they can be resistant to treatment. Some plantar warts are small, rounded, solitary lesions, while others involve large patches of skin from roughly two to four inches across.

Plantar warts can be difficult to treat because of their location on the bottom of the foot. The skin on the bottom of the foot is twice as thick as the skin on other parts of the body. This thicker skin allows the wart to penetrate deeper and prevents topical medications from reaching all of the wart.

Warts can also be somewhat unpredictable. They can take weeks or months to resolve, sometimes spreading even during aggressive treatment. And they can disappear on their own, without treatment. Treating plantar warts takes patience and persistence and sometimes requires changing or combining different treatment methods. For these reasons, always have a doctor evaluate a suspected wart before treating it yourself.

Do not pick at warts with your fingers. The viral tissue can embed itself in the skin around the fingernails and cause warts on the fingers as well.

Most over-the-counter wart treatments contain salicylic acid. Liquid wart treatments contain 17 percent of the acid, and medicated patches contain 40 percent. For warts resistant to over-the-counter treatment, your doctor may use more aggressive treatments. Such treatments include removing the wart with laser treatment, prescribing medications, or freezing (and killing) the wart with liquid nitrogen. A study published in 2002 , however, found that simply covering a wart with a patch of duct tape was as effective as treating it with liquid nitrogen.[7]

Recently, a refrigerant spray has become available for treating warts without a prescription. The treatment may be able to remove warts on the hands or tops of the feet by "freezing" them, but it is unlikely that it is strong enough to kill plantar warts. Relatively expensive, the kits are probably less effective than other treatments. And they can damage healthy skin if misused.

For reasons we don't understand, children and teenagers tend to be able to resolve warts more quickly than adults. It is suspected that, as it ages, the immune system becomes less effective at fending off the virus that causes warts. It is not unusual for plantar warts to persist even after years of aggressive treatment.

Calluses and corns

Calluses and corns are thick patches of skin. Calluses on top of or between the toes are often referred to as corns. In this section, the term *callus* is used to refer to both corns and calluses. Calluses are often confused with warts, but a wart is caused by a virus entering the skin. A callus is caused by excessive pressure or friction. A callus usually appears as a patch of hard, dry skin that is the same color as the skin around it. Unlike a wart, skin lines can be seen in the skin of a callus. Calluses aren't always easily identified and treated. If, after one or two weeks of self-treatment, a suspected callus has not improved, you should have it evaluated by a medical professional. Some skin lesions can mimic a callus. And sometimes a callus can obscure an injury to the skin or underlying structures.

Remember that calluses are always caused by pressure or friction. They do not arise randomly. They will only go away if the source of pressure or friction is addressed. Skin defends itself from injury by producing thicker layers, but those thicker layers can then become irritated and painful if the pressure or friction that created them persists. Pumicing, trimming, cutting, or even surgically removing a callus will not lead to long-term relief if you don't stop the pressure or friction that caused it in the first place.

A number of conditions can cause pressure or friction sufficient enough to form a callus. They include the atrophy (shrinking) of soft tissues, deformities, bony prominences (bumps), and pressure from s that are too small or too narrow.

Calluses on the toes are often caused by changes in the alignment of the toes, which occurs with hammertoes and bunions. Changes in alignment make the toes rub together or against a shoe, creating friction. Wearing shoes that are too narrow for your feet can also cause calluses on the toes, especially between the toes. To treat calluses on the toes you must first minimize or eliminate the rubbing. This can be done by padding the toes with gel or foam toe spacers or, even better, by wearing shoes that fit properly.

Though uncommon, calluses can break down into open sores or ulcers. They can also become infected. Have your primary care doctor or podiatrist look at any callus that becomes red, painful, or bleeds as soon as possible.

Calluses on the bottom of the foot are most often found on the ball of the foot, or forefoot. These calluses are usually caused by excessive pressure on the forefoot bones. This pressure can develop when the protective fat pads on the bottom of the foot shrink or when hammertoes cause the metatarsal bones to press down against the bottom of the foot. Arthritis can also cause calluses on the forefoot, because it limits joint motion and can lead to the development of bony protrusions. Most forefoot calluses can be addressed by simply distributing pressure in the shoe through modifications to the insoles. (See the chapter on insoles for more information.)

Calluses on the ends of the toes, especially the middle three toes, are common. These calluses are often caused by hammertoes. The contracting toes begin to bear weight on the tips instead of the bottoms of the toes, resulting in calluses. Using crest pads or toe splints (see the chapter on toe conditions) can help align the toes and minimize the formation of calluses.

Underlying injuries

The pressure that causes calluses can also cause pressure-related injuries to the skin, soft tissues, joints, and bones beneath them. Places on the foot that stick out, such as bony prominences and joints, are common locations for calluses and, therefore, for pressure-related injuries. Redness that surrounds a painful callus, for example, can be a symptom of bursitis. Bursitis is an inflammation of the bursa, or fluid-filled sac, that lies between the skin and the bone. Bursitis of the feet is most commonly seen on the tops of hammertoes or the sides of bunions. Redness around the callus can also be a sign of underlying infection, so it should not be ignored.

Pressure on the joints of the bottom of the foot can cause capsulitis, or inflammation of the joint capsule (the tissue that surrounds the joint). Capsulitis is most common in the second toe joint of the forefoot and is often seen in combination with hammertoes and bunions.

Some calluses have irregularly shaped areas of dark red or purple. This is often a sign that the pressure on the underlying soft tissue has caused some bleeding under the skin. Although usually painless, the bleeding is an early warning that the callus could progress to an open sore or ulcer. Discolored calluses are especially worrisome for those with diabetes, neuropathy, or circulation disorders. They should be examined by a podiatrist or general practitioner.

Cracking skin

Very large, thick calluses can occasionally develop on the feet. They are most commonly found around the heel or under the big toe joint. Occasionally they become so thick and dry that the skin cannot stretch when weight is placed on the foot. When this happens, the skin cracks open, resulting in bleeding and painful fissures that are vulnerable to infection and difficult to heal. See a doctor if you have fissured skin that is painful or bleeding, especially if you also have poor circulation, diabetes, or a history of poor healing.

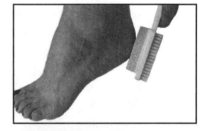

If the fissured skin is not painful or bleeding, you can treat it yourself by following these daily steps:

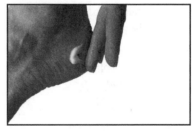

- Wash the skin with warm soap and water.
- Use a pumice stone to gently reduce the thick callus over time.
- Apply an exfoliating cream.

After washing the callus, gently rub it with a pumice stone. Then apply an exfoliating cream.

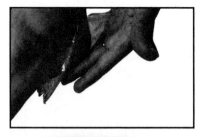

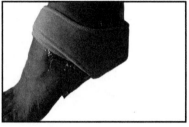

For stubborn cases, try wrapping the moisturized skin overnight.

For persistent or severe cracks, treating twice a day may be necessary. For the most stubborn cases, apply the lotion and then cover the cracked skin with a plastic wrap or a commercially available heel moisturizing neoprene wrap. Sleeping with the wrap in place for two to three consecutive nights can work wonders.

Some over-the-counter "skin glue" products have recently become available. They are applied to the cracked skin, helping seal out infection and promote healing. Any crack that has not healed within one week of self-treatment should be seen by a doctor.

Pressure ulcers

If untreated, corns and calluses—and sometimes blisters—can become open sores, or ulcers. If the pressure that caused the callus persists, eventually the skin and soft tissue beneath the callus can break down, resulting in an open sore. These sores are often referred to as pressure ulcers. They can masquerade as painful (or sometimes painless) red calluses. Pressure ulcers on the feet are a concern because they can easily become infected. They are also often difficult to heal because the pressure decreases blood flow. Walking or wearing shoes can prolong the healing process.

The absence of pain is not always a good sign. A significant complicating factor of many pressure ulcers is the inability to feel the pain they cause. Sufferers may not even be aware that an ulcer is forming on their feet. Those with a "high pain threshold" or decreased sensation should visually inspect their feet daily.

Like calluses, ulcers occur in areas where the skin is subjected to excessive pressure or friction. This is why most pressure ulcers are found on the bottom of the forefoot. People with diabetes, poor circulation, and numbness in the feet are especially vulnerable to pressure ulcers. Poor hygiene, poor nutrition, and poorly fitting shoes can also be contributing factors. But sometimes even wearing slippers or going barefoot around the house can lead to pressure ulcers.

Seed corns (porokeratosis)

Some calluses can develop a hard center much like a seed or small stone in the skin. This type of callus is known as a seed corn or, more formally, porokeratosis. Seed corns are especially painful and difficult to treat, and they can be easily mistaken for plantar warts. It is best to have these calluses evaluated and treated by a podiatrist.

Three steps to callus care

The safest and surest self-care for calluses involves the three following steps:

(1) **Relieve the pressure on the callus.** First and most importantly, you should relieve the pressure causing the callus by using padding, stretching or replacing your shoes, or modifying the insoles in your shoes.

(2) **Reduce the thickness of the callus.** Regular, gentle use of a pumice stone is safer than shaving the callus with sharp cutting tools. Rubbing the callus with a pumice stone for one minute after bathing three to four times per week is an effective way for most people to reduce the thickness of a callus.

(3) **Soften and moisturize.** Apply exfoliating lotion or cream to the callus once or twice daily. (Do not apply lotions or creams between toes unless directed by a medical professional.)

Relieve the pressure

You can relieve pressure on your feet by using pads, modifying your shoes, or applying digital sleeves (toe splints). For people who have difficulty reaching their feet, permanently adjusting a shoe is the easiest and most effective way of relieving pressure on a callus. What's more, pads applied to a shoe adhere better than ones applied to the skin, so you don't have to reapply them quite so often. One other consideration: applying adhesive pads directly to the foot can irritate the skin. This potential irritation can be avoided by applying the pad to the shoe instead. The most versatile padding is adhesive moleskin, a product that is found in most pharmacies and can be cut to the necessary size and shape.

Shoe modifications to relieve pressure

By some estimates, one out of four people would benefit from modifying their footwear. For those with foot pain or difficult to fit feet, that percentage is surely higher. Some very simple shoe modifications, such as stretching or padding, to relieve pressure points can have tremendous benefits. A podiatrist or certified pedorthist can provide invaluable advice in this regard.

Shoes with removable insoles are best for making modifications. Often, after the shoes have been worn for a few weeks, an imprint of the foot can be seen on the insole. This imprint makes it easier to determine the best location to place padding. Because many insoles compress in areas of pressure, placing a pad for a painful forefoot callus is done simply by finding the dented area of the insole and padding around it—*not* on it.

Relieving pressure with moleskin is achieved by applying shaped pads cut to size. Horseshoe pads, donut pads, or parallel strips of padding around the painful area work very well in distributing pressure away from the affected area.

When it is not obvious where to pad the shoe, there is a simple trick for locating the proper area and applying the padding:

- Mark the painful area on the skin with a dot of lipstick and then step into the shoe without a sock.
- Make sure the skin contacts the shoe by pressing on the shoe with your fingers. When the shoe is removed, the pressure area will be obvious by the lipstick mark.
- Place padding around (not on) the lipstick mark.

Placing padding directly on the skin can be done periodically or in an emergency to temporarily offload pressure on a callus. But for long-term relief, it is best to pad the shoes instead. Not only will the padding last longer, but you are less likely to develop a skin rash or tear the skin. Unless directed by a doctor, you should not use any adhesive products on your skin if you have diabetes, a circulation disorder, or skin that is especially fragile, sensitive, or thin.

Shoes that do not have removable insoles can also be modified, but it is much more difficult to do so. As a general rule, shoes that don't have removable insoles aren't going to be as cushioned or supportive as those that do. If it is necessary to purchase a more supportive insole to add to the shoe, that insole will fit better into the shoe if the original insole is first removed. But simple modifications can be made with commercially available adhesive pads to just about any shoe if necessary.

There is also a commercially available forefoot sleeve that looks like a sock for the forefoot. The slip-on fabric sleeve has a large gel pad in the forefoot that can offer great cushioning. The forefoot sleeve works especially well when wearing slippers, sandals, or shoes that do not have adequate cushioning.

Padding and insoles to relieve pressure
There are a number of over-the-counter shoe padding products and insoles available and, frankly, many of them don't live up to their claims. For example, insoles are designed to protect the bottom of the feet and may be fitted for the full length of the foot or for the arch alone. Unfortunately, what you tend to find on the shelf are compromised products. By this I mean that the manufacturer has compromised the ability of the product to relieve pressure in order to make it more attractive and marketable to the consumer. Manufacturers of footcare products know that women suffer more foot pain than men and are

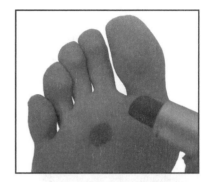

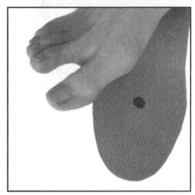

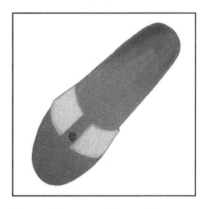

To see where to pad your shoe to relieve pressure on a callus, mark the painful area with lipstick, then transfer the mark to your shoe.

33

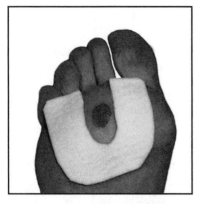

For temporary relief, a horseshoe-shaped pad can sometimes be applied directly to the skin around a callus to relieve pressure. But it is better to apply the padding to the shoe or insole.

more likely to seek treatment for their foot pain than men, so they try to attract women to their products by making them soft and thin enough to fit into women's dress shoes. These products are less dense and cushioned than needed to be effective. Beware of very thin or very soft padding and insoles that claim to cushion the foot. They usually won't. If a padding or insole doesn't appear capable of supporting your full weight or absorbing impact without compressing flat, then look for something better.

Sometimes, no amount of modification can fix a shoe, and it's best simply to eliminate the source of the pain. Instead of trying to pad a tight, unsupportive shoe, replace it with a more supportive, better fitting (even if less stylish) shoe—at least until the foot problem improves. If you have tried and failed to find relief with over-the-counter products, see a podiatrist.

Here are some recommendations for quality, over-the-counter products for modifying footwear:

Moleskin is a type of padding made from cotton, synthetic material, or wool. It has an adhesive backing and can be cut to any shape and applied to the inside of shoes or to the feet. It is found in the footcare section of most pharmacies. Moleskin comes in different thicknesses and densities. The softer types are less effective at distributing pressure and are less durable. When applied to shoes or insoles, moleskin should be replaced or layered as it compresses or shifts.

Wool felt is a medical-grade padding that has an adhesive backing and is very durable, especially when compared to some brands of moleskin. It is not available in most stores, but it can be found on the Internet. Wool felt can be custom cut and applied directly to the insides of shoes, insoles, or, temporarily, the foot.

Metatarsal pads are rounded pads designed to decrease pressure on the ball of the foot by increasing pressure at the end of the arch. When properly placed (at the end of the arch just before the ball of the foot), they can relieve pain from forefoot calluses. There are so many different types of metatarsal pads available over the counter that consumers can be easily confused. The best metatarsal pads are those made from wool felt. They should feel firm. Foam, gel, thin, and flat metatarsal pads usually do not work effectively. The Hapad company makes wool metatarsal pads that are of medical-grade quality and effectiveness.

When padding the inside of a shoe to prevent forefoot calluses, place the padding around the point of pressure and not directly on it. Padding around the callus "offloads" the pressure (moves it away). Padding placed directly on the pressure point only increases the pressure on the callus.

Aperture pads are donut- or horseshoe-shaped pads that can be placed around a painful callus. Some are available precut, while others can be custom-cut from moleskin. Donut- or horseshoe-shaped pads work well for relieving pressure on the callus. Foam aperture pads work best on the tops of toes (to protect calluses or hammertoes) or the sides of the feet (to protect bunions) but do not work as well for painful areas on the bottoms of the feet. An insole with a wool moleskin pad will protect the bottom of the feet better and last longer than foam.

Digital pads come in the form of sleeves, adhesive donut-shaped pads, or toe spacers and are made of silicone gel, foam, or felt. Toe sleeves slip over and wrap the toe. Adhesive felt or foam can be applied to the skin around a painful callus, and spacers can be placed between the toes to relieve pressure. It is important to avoid shoes that put pressure on the toes.

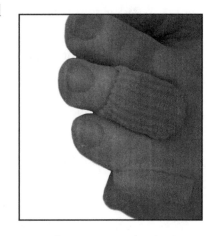

A toe sleeve protects the third toe, while a foam spacer relieves pressure between the fourth and fifth toes.

Buy padding or insoles that are durable and dense. Do the "pinch test": If you can easily compress the padding or insole between your thumb and forefinger, there is no way that it can hold up to the impact of daily walking, and you should choose another product. As a general rule, avoid thick foam or thin gel pads and insoles.

Insoles are probably the most effective way to treat many foot disorders. Until recently there were few choices for insoles. Now, some stores carry ten to fifteen different types. Shoe padding products include moleskin, gel cushions, heel cups, arch pads and metatarsal pads (rounded pads designed to protect the forefoot). Insoles can be made from foam, plastic, gel, or fabric. The selection can actually be quite overwhelming. Insoles are most effective for treating and preventing calluses on the bottoms of feet because they can be modified to relieve pressure and they can be moved from one pair of shoes to another.

Shoe changes for toe calluses

Calluses on the tops of toes are most often caused by hammertoes. The bent toe takes up more room in the shoe and rubs against the inside of the shoe's toe box. Often, the small toe is squeezed by shoes that are too narrow or too pointed. This is especially true for women, as women's fashionable shoes often are more narrow and pointed than men's.

If you have painful hammertoes with calluses, try changing to shoes that have additional depth or a more rounded shape to give your toes more room. A hammertoe splint can also reduce the contracting of the toe that contributes to the callus. In severe cases that do not respond to shoes changes, splints, or other types of self-care, it may be necessary to correct hammertoes surgically.

Reduce the thickness

After addressing the cause of a callus, the next step is to do some basic skin care. A pumice stone, emery board, or similar sanding device can be used to gently remove some of the thick, dry layers of a callus. Often, it is helpful to use an exfoliating cream or lotion in addition to pumicing.

The skin is softest just after a bath or shower, so this is the ideal time to use the pumice stone. By lightly rubbing the pumice stone over the callus for one to two minutes after bathing over the course of several days, the callus can be gradually reduced. This is a much safer way of removing skin than using razor blades or callus knives. Keep in mind, however, that the callus has a protective function. Removing too much dry skin may cause a sore to develop because the skin no longer has the thicker, firmer skin of the callus to protect it from pressure or friction. This is why it is always important to remove the source of the pressure or friction before doing any other kind of treatment.

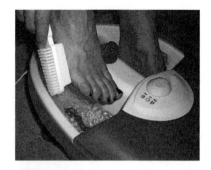

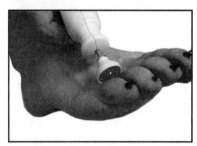

Soften and lubricate

After pumicing a callus, apply an exfoliating cream or lotion. The exfoliating ingredient will further reduce the callus and soften the remaining skin so that the next pumice treatment will be more effective.

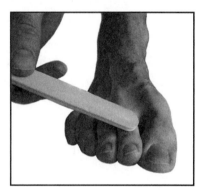

The most effective over-the-counter exfoliating lotions contain salicylic, uric, or lactic acids. These gentle acids work by dissolving the hard, dry layers of the callus. Emollients in these creams and lotions moisturize the callus and the skin around it. For more stubborn calluses or dry skin, there are prescription-strength exfoliating lotions.

A pumice stone or power rotary tool with a sanding disk can be used to decrease the thickness of a callus. An emery board works well on small calluses on the tops or sides of the toes.

A word of caution: exfoliating lotions—both over the counter and prescription—do have side effects. These include redness, burning, and sun sensitivity. Use exfoliating lotions only as directed. Skin that is not dry or callused is especially irritated by the acids in these lotions. Skin irritation usually resolves once you stop applying the lotion, but if side effects persist, consult a doctor. Once the callus is satisfactorily treated, periodic treatments may be necessary to control the callus.

How *not* to treat a callus

There are several things you should *not* do to treat a callus:

- Do *not* treat a callus until you are certain that it is a callus. If there is doubt, see a podiatrist.
- Do *not* attempt to cut out a callus. "Bathroom surgery" can result in injury and infection.

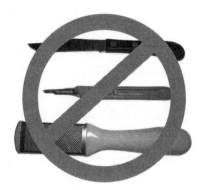

- Do *not* use metal callus files that resemble cheese graters. They can gouge and shred the skin.
- Avoid medicated corn pads. Medicated corn pads are dangerous because the "medication" is actually a strong acid, which can burn the skin and cause an open sore. Often, medicated corn pads also burn healthy skin around calluses.

Slow and steady treatment methods combined with pressure relief are the safest ways to treat calluses.

Skin Care Myths

Many people believe that white socks are better for the feet than dark socks. This thinking may actually have more to do with fabric than color, since we tend to associate white socks with cotton and we tend to think of cotton as being more natural and healthier than other fabrics. But the truth is that cotton blends and certain new synthetic fabrics keep feet drier and cooler in the summer and warmer in the winter. This is important, since dry feet are less prone to blisters, infections, athlete's foot, and foul odor. DuPont makes a fabric called CoolMax that is excellent at wicking moisture from the skin. There are several other foot-friendly brands as well, including Smart Wool, New Balance, and Wigwam.

Another common belief is that it is good to soak your feet in water. Like many things, soaking the feet can be good—if done in moderation. But excessive foot soaking can overhydrate the skin, weakening it and making it more vulnerable to injury. Paradoxically, excessive soaking or bathing, particularly if soap is used, removes the natural oils of the skin that help retain moisture, causing the feet to become too dry.

3

Nail Care

One of the most common reasons people go to a podiatrist is because of problems with their toenails. The incidence of such problems increases as we age. And even though most age-related changes to the toenails do not cause pain or create a health issue, many people are embarrassed by the way their nails look. Dry, thick, discolored, and misshapen nails simply make people self-conscious.

Caring for toenails can be difficult, even intimidating—especially trimming them—if they are thick, tough, or painful. Medical conditions can also complicate matters. For example, if you are taking a blood-thinning medication such as Coumadin (warfarin), you must be cautious when caring for your nails (or any skin condition) because of the risk of bleeding. If you have arthritis in your hands or back, you may find it difficult to reach your feet or use clippers. Other challenges include visual impairment or decreased feeling in the hands or feet.

This chapter, then, is written with the knowledge that the responsibility for nail care often falls to spouses, other family members, or caregivers. The decision to seek professional care for nails should be based on overall health, skin and nail conditions, and other limiting or complicating medical conditions. If in doubt, talk with your primary doctor or a podiatrist.

Nail hygiene

Good nail care starts with good foot hygiene. Cleansing and caring for the feet on a daily basis is important for minimizing the risk of infections, athlete's foot, dry skin, and nail problems. Toenail and skin problems tend to be much worse in people who have poor foot hygiene. Accumulating dirt, moisture, fungus, and bacteria contribute to odors, skin changes, and discoloration and thickening of the toenails.

Basic foot hygiene consists of washing the feet with soap and water, drying the skin thoroughly, and using powders, lotions, or topical medications as needed. Treating athlete's foot quickly and diligently is especially important to minimize the risk of fungal nails.

Good foot hygiene, finally, requires good shoes and socks. Old shoes and unwashed socks can harbor and promote bacteria, fungus, and odor. Wear a fresh pair of socks each day. Throw away old, smelly shoes.

Nail anatomy

The nail is made up of a hard layer of a substance produced by cells located under the skin at the base of the nail. The nail grows over what is called the nail bed. The thin layer of tissue at the edge of the nail as it meets the skin is called the cuticle. A healthy nail is smooth and clear. It should be firmly attached to the nail bed, and it should grow a little over an inch a year.

Nail care

Most people need to trim their toenails about every six to eight weeks. As the body ages, though, the nails grow more slowly. Older adults may only need to trim their toenails at intervals of three to six months. How long you go between nail trimmings is a matter of personal preference. In general, though, keeping the nails too short (so short that they hurt after trimming or become ingrown) can cause more problems than allowing them

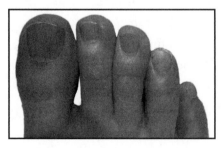

Healthy nails trimmed to the proper length.

to grow longer. However, excessively long nails can also become ingrown and are more vulnerable to injury and infection.

Nail care, when done properly and regularly, will help maintain the health and integrity of the nails and the surrounding skin. Investing the time and energy in good footcare practices minimizes the risks of nail and skin problems. The following sections describe the basic steps necessary for good toenail care.

Nail tools

As with any task, the job of caring for your nails is much easier if you have the proper tools. Of course, the basic tool you will need is a clipper. The traditional toenail clipper is a larger version of the fingernail clipper. A small toenail clipper will work well on healthy nails of normal thickness. Larger, pliers-shaped clippers are better for trimming thick nails. Those with a spring mechanism tend to have the best cutting power. The cost of the clipper will vary according to its quality. The more expensive clippers can be sharpened. Less expensive clippers should be replaced when they become dull.

Emery boards or fine nail files are handy nail care tools. They can smooth rough nail edges, round off nail corners and, in some cases, be used to reduce the thickness of problem nails. (As noted previously, emery boards also work well for reducing the thickness of calluses between the toes.) Most emery boards and nail files are inexpensive and can be purchased at any pharmacy.

Power pedicure kits are relatively new to the nonprofessional footcare market. They

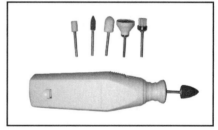
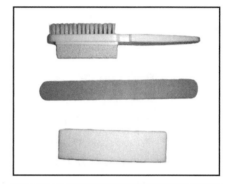
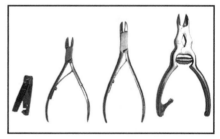

Selecting the proper nail instrument is an important part of nail care.
Top: A brush with a pumice stone; an emery board; and pumice stone
Middle: A power rotary device
Bottom: Assorted nail clippers

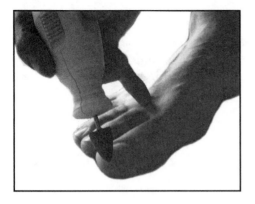

You can use a power rotary tool to buff down overly thick nails and smooth out rough edges.

can range in price from twenty dollars to more than one hundred dollars. Pedicure kits contain a power rotary device with attachments for thinning, grinding, and buffing the nails. Some have an attachment for treating calluses as well. The kits are especially helpful for trimming thick nails that are too difficult to cut with a clipper. If you use a rotary device, be very careful not to injure the nail, nail bed, and the skin around the nail. Moistening nails before treatment will help to decrease the heat that tends to build up during the thinning process. Moving the device back and forth over the nail so that heat does not build up in one area can also reduce the risk of injury. For extremely thick toenails, thinning and grinding is more safely done over the course of multiple treatments. Because grinding the toenails can create an aerosol of fungal and nail dust that can cause lung or eye problems, you may want to seek out a professional with proper safety equipment to perform this nail care service for you.

Nail trimming

The best time to trim the nails is just after a bath or shower. (Some people prefer to soak their feet for fifteen to twenty minutes before trimming.) The moisture helps to soften the nails, making them easier to trim than dry nails. (Regular use of topical nail solutions, discussed in another section, also helps to soften dry, hard nails.) To trim your nails, begin by gently placing the lower jaw of the clipper against the skin under the nail and the upper jaw above the nail. This will push the skin away from the cutting surface. Slowly squeeze the jaws together before cutting to make sure there is no pain. If there is pain, reposition the jaws. (Never cut without knowing exactly what you've grasped between the jaws of the clipper.) Cut the nail straight across, leaving a little nail protruding over the edge of the nail bed and rounding the nail corners slightly. Use an emery board, nail file, or rotary tool to gently smooth and round the corners. Do not cut the nails too short or trim aggressively into the corners, as both can lead to ingrown nails and infections.

There is a common misconception that cuticles are an unnecessary part of the nail and are best removed. This is simply not true. The cuticle helps to seal the edge of the nail where it meets the skin. It is an important barrier to debris and infection. It should not be removed.

If you have, or suspect that you have, a fungal infection in one or more of your nails, it is wise to use separate instruments for the healthy nails to avoid cross-contamination. Simply washing the tools does not guarantee that the fungus will be removed.

If a toenail is persistently painful or difficult to trim, you may want to consult a podiatrist. A podiatrist can demonstrate trimming techniques that may alleviate the pain or, if necessary, treat the nail medically. Most nail conditions can be treated painlessly. Only a tiny percentage of people will ever need to have part or all of a nail removed to fix a toenail problem.

Can you reach your feet? The most common reason I hear from patients who have problems trimming their nails is that they cannot reach their feet. If you do not have a family member who can trim your toenails for you, you may have to rely on a podiatrist or footcare nurse.

Professional nail care services

There is no substitute for expert care. Podiatrists are nail care experts. Their education and training make them your best option for diagnosing and treating all nail conditions. Some podiatrists make regular visits to senior centers, community centers, and homes, in addition to keeping their regular office hours. But there are other nail care professionals who can assist with nail care as well.

Footcare nurses specialize in nail and skin care. Many local senior centers offer access to footcare nurses. Footcare nurses typically do not accept health insurance, but their rates for trimming calluses and toenails tend to be very reasonable. Footcare nurses can also assess foot and nail conditions and make referrals to a podiatrist as necessary.

For most people, a reputable nail salon is a viable option for basic foot and nail care. However, if you have a circulation disorder, diabetes, or numbness in your feet, you should avoid nail salons and see a doctor or other health care provider instead. If you do decide to visit a nail salon, check it out carefully first. Ask the nail technician if he or she uses sterile instruments and cleans the foot basin (not just changes the water) between customers. If not, find another salon. Even when you find a good nail technician, consider bringing your own nail instruments to the salon to minimize the risk of infection. Make sure the technician trims nails properly and does not remove the cuticles.

Paying for Professional Nail Care Services

If you have diabetes, a circulation disorder, a nerve disorder, or a history of limb ulcers or amputation, you may qualify for medical nail and callus care under Medicare guidelines. Ask your insurance provider, primary care doctor, or podiatrist whether you qualify for coverage. Even if you have to pay for services yourself, it is often much safer and, in the long run, more cost-effective to have a podiatrist treat your feet. You could benefit from just one or two nail care visits a year.

Common toenail conditions

Certain common toenail conditions can complicate the care of your nails. Most of us will experience changes in the shape, texture, and color of our nails as we age. These changes are often no more than a nuisance. But sometimes they can result in pain or infection. In addition to signs of aging, changes in the toenails can also be symptoms of systemic disease, so they should not be taken lightly or ignored, especially if they affect both the hands and the feet.

Age-related changes in toenails

Over the course of a lifetime, the toenails take quite a beating. Remember, we take five to ten thousand steps a day, often while wearing hot, confining footwear. The toenails are subjected to much more daily abuse than fingernails, and confining them in shoes for extended periods of time makes them even more vulnerable to injury and infection.

It is not uncommon for toenails that have been injured or subjected to constant pressure to become thick and painful over time. This can happen to one or several nails. The nails of the big toe and the small toe are usually the first to show age-related changes, because they tend to bear the brunt of shoe pressure. Most problems caused by age-related nail changes respond well to good foot hygiene, proper nail and skin care, and the use of topical medications.

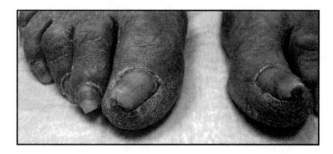

Common nail changes are seen above: thickness, discoloration, and altered nail shape.

As noted above, your nails tend to grow more slowly as you age. The good news is that you may not have to trim your nails so often. The bad news is that your nails can become more vulnerable to fungal infection and slower to heal from injuries. One theory on why older people are more likely to have fungal infections of the toenails is that the slower growing nail allows fungus living on the skin to advance up and under the end of the nail and infect the nail from the bottom up. Basically, the fungus advances faster than the growing nail can "push" it away.

Changes in nail color

When nails change color, they most commonly turn yellow, but they can also appear brown, gray, blue, or red. Color changes can affect the whole nail or only part of it. In some cases the color changes are not in the nail at all but in the skin under the nail. Sometimes, a change in the color of the toenails can be cause by an injury. A discoloration of this sort usually grows out with the nail and is gradually trimmed away with routine nail care. The discoloration can, however, take up to a year to resolve. The yellowing associated with fungus often moves from the end of the nail back toward the base of the nail as the fungal infection advances. This process can occur very slowly over the course of several years. Yellowing of the nails sometimes improves or even resolves with topical or oral antifungal treatment.

Colored lines can also occur in the nails. A white line across the nail from side-to-side is commonly called a Mee's line. This line often affects more than one nail, but it can occur in just one. The line advances with the growing nail and may be a symptom of congestive heart failure, the effects of chemotherapy, or a systemic insult. Bands of white lines that disappear when the nail is compressed are called Muehrcke's lines. Unlike Mee's lines, Muehrcke's lines do not advance as the nail grows. Muehrcke's lines can be caused by liver disease or malnutrition.

White lines in the nail that are oriented lengthwise (instead of across the nail from one side to the other) are usually of no significance and are likely just a result of minor trauma to the nail or of the normal aging process. Occasionally they are accompanied by lengthwise ridges in the nail as well.

Red or brown lines that are oriented along the length of the nail (not side-to-side) are often splinter hemorrhages. They result from rupture of small blood vessels. They may be caused by trauma, psoriasis, or endocarditis. If they are accompanied by fever and similar changes to the skin around the nail, they should be evaluated by a doctor.

People with darker skin often have dark nail discoloration or lines. While this is most often an incidental finding, it can make it more difficult to distinguish benign conditions from more serious conditions.

There are several causes for changes in nail color that need to be addressed by a general practitioner or podiatrist. These causes include bacterial infections, circulation changes (usually decreased circulation), poor nutrition, and drug reactions. Certain diseases, including skin cancer, psoriasis, kidney disease, rheumatoid arthritis, and diabetes, can also cause nail discoloration. If you suspect any of these causes, seek the advice of a doctor.

Unless you've injured your nail, you should see a physician if a nail darkens in order to rule out certain types of benign or malignant skin lesions that can develop under the nail.

Bleeding under the nail

Black, purple, or blue color changes to the nail after a nail injury usually mean there is bleeding under the nail. Bleeding under the nail is commonly caused by dropping something heavy on the toenail or stubbing the toe against a hard object. It can also be caused by wearing a tight pair of shoes or having a thick nail. If the nail is not painful, it does not need to be treated. Typically, a damaged nail will loosen over the course of several weeks or months until it separates completely. Gradually, a new nail will grow out to replace the old one. In fact, the injured nail is often "pushed off" as the new nail grows underneath it. It usually takes eight to ten months for the new nail to completely grow out over the nail bed. If you have an injured nail that is loosening from the nail bed, trim it so that it does not catch on your socks or sheets. Nails with loose edges can also be covered with a bandage or medical tape to prevent further injury.

If the nail is painful and there is noticeable redness or swelling, the blood may need to be drained. Draining often offers dramatic and immediate pain relief as the pressure under the nail is reduced. A medical professional should perform this procedure to avoid further injury and infection.

Changes in nail shape

There are many reasons why the shape of the toenails may change over time, including hereditary factors, injuries, changes in circulation, and fungal infections. The most common change is a thickening of the nail. In the most advanced cases, nails can become more than half an inch thick. Other changes in shape include curving, clubbing, and "spoon-shaped" nails.

Thickening of the toenail is often caused by a fungal infection. Fortunately for those who are vulnerable to thickening of the nails, a thorough nail treatment, done one to four times annually by a podiatrist, can control the problem.

Curving usually occurs at the corners of the nails and can lead to ingrown nails, nails with a peak at the center, or nails that become tubular in shape. A curved nail is probably the most difficult to trim and tends to become progressively more curved with time.

"Clubbing" refers to nails that have a bulbous shape, and appears in the fingers as well as the toes of affected individuals. The nail broadens and bulges as it curves downward around the end of the toe. It also becomes thin and rubbery and can separate from the nail bed. Clubbing is often an indication of heart or lung disease.

Spoon-shaped nails loosen and curve upwards at the ends of the toes and are thin, dry, and whitish in color. They usually indicate a systemic condition, such as iron deficiency anemia, systemic lupus, or Raynaud's disease/phenomenon.

Brittle nails, ridging, and pitting

Changes in the texture of the nails often accompany changes in the color and shape of the nails and may reflect the additional side effects of a fungal infection, systemic condition, or poor nutrition. Common changes in texture include brittleness, pitting, and ridging. Brittleness can become so severe that nails chip, crack, break off, or loosen from the nail bed. "Pitting" refers to the appearance of tiny pits in the nail; it is most commonly caused by psoriatic arthritis. There is no treatment for pitting. Ridges in the nail are often caused by trauma, but can develop after a serious illness. They represent a temporary interruption in normal nail growth. Changes in the texture of the nails can be treated with topical medications, but first the systemic cause of the changes should be identified and treated by a physician.

Loose toenails

Loose toenails are a cause for concern because they can catch and tear away from the nail bed. Most often caused by trauma, they can also result from fungal infection, poor circulation or nutrition, or hypothyroidism. It is best to trim a loose nail as short as is comfortably possible. The shorter nail may be less attractive, but it will also be less vulnerable to injury. Protecting the loose nail with an adhesive bandage or piece of tape is also a good idea. After the loose nail has been trimmed away or falls off on its own, you may want to treat the nail bed with a topical antifungal daily until the new nail has advanced to the end of the toe. This can take up to ten months. Treating the nail with an antifungal will help to avoid some of the nail changes that can occur after a nail has loosened or fallen off.

Ingrown toenails

When a toenail starts to curve downward, it can begin to press into the skin, becoming ingrown and causing pain, bleeding, and infection. Ingrown nails have several causes, including pressure from shoes, heredity, improper nail trimming, previous injuries, and fungal infections. And sometimes there is no identifiable cause of ingrown nails other than abnormal growth.

Thin, or bendable, toenails are prone to curving inward and becoming ingrown (as are fungal nails). In fact, thin toenails can sometimes fold in at the corners so severely that they take on a tubular shape. It is possible to make curving nails and ingrown curving nails worse by continually picking at them or cutting them too short. (This is true for any ingrown nail.) Bendable nails are best evaluated by a podiatrist for the most helpful course of treatment.

To prevent ingrown nails, allow the nail edge to grow out instead of cutting into the corner. If this method fails to prevent or heal the ingrown nail, seek the opinion of a podiatrist. For persistent or recurrent ingrown nails, minor surgery may be recommended.

Surgery for ingrown nails

Persistent ingrown nails that cause frequent pain or infections may need to be treated with a simple and relatively painless nail procedure performed by a podiatrist on an outpatient basis. Some people mistakenly believe that ingrown toenails have to be completely removed. This is usually not the case. Often, an ingrown nail edge can be removed under local anesthetic and the base of the nail treated so that that edge does not form again as the nail grows out. Patients walk out of the office with a light

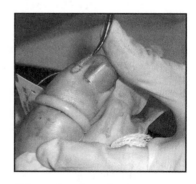

Often, the edge of an ingrown nail can be removed under local anesthetic, as shown above.

Patients have come to my clinic after suffering for years with a painful toenail. They were afraid to have the toe looked at because they thought the only treatment was some barbaric and painful surgical procedure. The truth is, it is rare that a nail has to be completely removed. Often, just the edge of the nail needs to be removed in a simple procedure with little discomfort. Most people say this discomfort is less than what they were already tolerating from the nail, and if they had known it was so easy, they would have come in much earlier.

dressing on the toe and are usually able to go about their normal activities with minimal discomfort.

Bathroom surgery is never recommended for ingrown toenails—or any other ailment, for that matter. Fearing painful nail surgery, some people will resort to self-surgery, using razors, knives, or even scissors to dig out painful nails. But an office-based procedure is less painful, significantly reduces the risk of infection and injury, and is much more effective, often providing permanent relief.

Painful, bleeding toenails

The inflammation and pressure from an ingrown nail border can, occasionally, cause a red, painful area that bleeds easily next to the nail. Called a pyogenic granuloma, it is essentially a capillary bed that has enlarged and raised above the skin. In addition to the pain and bleeding it causes, a pyogenic granuloma can also invite infection. It should be treated in a clinical setting as soon as possible. If you cannot see a doctor right away, keep the area bandaged until you can.

Questionable Ingrown Nail Treatments

There is simply no magical topical medication that can heal and correct an ingrown nail. Over-the-counter topical medications may temporarily decrease pain, but they do nothing to address the underlying nail condition. Popular wisdom has suggested that tucking cotton under the edge of an ingrown nail or cutting a V-notch into the end of the nail will fix problem ingrown nails. There may be some benefit, but these techniques do not work well, especially as a permanent solution.

Ingrown nails and bacterial infection

Ingrown toenails can cause infections because they cut into the skin and allow bacteria to invade the tissue around the nail. The infection causes redness, swelling, and sometimes pustular drainage and bleeding. Minor infections can be treated by soaking the foot with the affected toe in warm, soapy water for ten to twenty minutes, followed by applying a topical antibiotic ointment or iodine and then bandaging the site. It is best to see a doctor if the signs of infection have not resolved after one or two days. He or she will clean the site, check for and remove sharp edges or broken nail fragments embedded in the flesh, and possibly prescribe an oral antibiotic.

Fungal nails

Probably the most common complaint regarding the toenails is fungal infection. The same fungus that causes athlete's foot can also cause changes to the toenails. This fungus lives on the skin and is usually kept in check by the immune system. Occasionally, however, it evades our immune system and penetrates the nail.

As the fungus advances under the toenail, it causes the color of the nail to change, as well as making it grow thicker and more brittle. Most complaints about fungal nails are directed at the unsightly appearance of the affected nails. But, for some, the toenails can start to hurt as they become thicker and more brittle. Fungal infections also produce debris under the nail that looks like dry, flaking skin. In some cases, infected nails loosen from the nail bed.

Some nail changes can mimic a fungal infection, which is why a suspected fungal infection should be evaluated by a podiatrist or dermatologist. Accurate diagnosis is important to ensure proper treatment. And the only true way a podiatrist can diagnose the presence of fungus with certainty is to order a lab test on a sample of the affected nail.

Who's at risk for fungal nails? There are some common traits that those with fungal toenail infections

I am often asked if nail fungus is easily spread. The answer is, it depends—on your immune system and other factors. I've seen patients who were married to partners with fungus in all ten toenails but who did not develop symptoms themselves. And then I've seen whole families affected by fungal nails. If you are prone to fungal infections in your nails, you must be especially diligent about your foot hygiene.

often share. It seems that those who often get athlete's foot and those whose feet tend to sweat profusely are more likely to get fungal toenails. Keeping the skin cool and dry and treating athlete's foot aggressively are important for minimizing toenail problems. Occasionally, fungal nails have a hereditary component. Some people are simply born more susceptible to fungal infections than others.

Treatment of fungal nails

Fungal toenails are notoriously hard to treat. Topical medications alone are not often effective. Most are unable to penetrate through the nail to completely eradicate the fungus living in the nail bed. The only topical antifungal nail treatment currently approved by the FDA is a medication called Penlac. Oral antifungal medications have a higher success rate at resolving the fungal infection. But studies suggest that after clearing the infection with a prescription oral medication, there is still a relatively high chance of reinfection.[8]

While nonprescription topical antifungal medications cannot cure fungal infections, they can help treat them. Antifungal topicals often slow the advancement of the fungus, improve the appearance of the nails, and soften the nails, making them easier to care for. Common over-the-counter antifungal medications include NonyX, FungiCare, and Mycocide. These medications should be applied twice daily to the far end of the nail while pointing the toes upward. Applying the medication with the toes pointed upward helps draw the medication under the nail.

Oral antifungal medications are available by prescription only. These medications are expensive, and health insurance plans often have strict requirements for prescription approval. For most people, Medicare does not cover the cost of oral antifungal medication for treating the toenails. Other insurers require that a lab confirm the infection, that the condition be causing pain, that more than one nail be infected, or that other conditions, such as diabetes or circulation disorders, also be present. Those with more serious symptoms or systemic conditions are more vulnerable to secondary bacterial infections caused by severe fungal nails.

Treating fungal toenails can be a frustrating experience. There is no quick or easy treatment. Diligently treating the nails twice daily with a topical medication for six to ten months may achieve only mild improvement. Even the most effective treatment—prescription oral medication—requires taking a pill daily for three to four consecutive months and up to eight additional months for a healthy nail to gradually replace the fungal nail.

Fungus thrives in dark, moist environments. Airing out shoes and opening them up to direct sunlight is a great way to kill the fungus that may be living inside.

In addition to using medications, addressing fungus that lives in the shoes is an important part of minimizing the risk of fungal nails, treating them, and preventing recurrence after treatment. A study conducted at the University of Minnesota found that throwing away old shoes and socks after toenails had improved resulted in less chance of reinfection.[9] While this might be expensive and difficult (most of us have shoes that are hard to part with), fungus accumulates in shoes over time (and socks to a lesser degree, as socks can be washed), increasing the risk of infection and reinfection. This risk is heightened for people who live in warm climates or who have feet that sweat a lot. Wear clean socks every day. You should change your socks several times a day when it is warm and if you have sweaty feet. Air out shoes and expose them to sunlight to minimize the dark, moist conditions in which fungi thrive.

If you have a fungal infection, you should be especially careful with nail-care instruments to decrease the risk of spreading the fungus to other nails. It is best to use two sets of instruments, especially nail clippers—one for the fungal nails and the other for the healthy nails. An third set should be used for care of the fingernails. Instruments used to treat fungal nails should be discarded following successful treatment.

Home remedies for fungal nails
Folklore, propagated by the Internet, is full of "sure-fire cures" for fungal nails. These home remedies include bleach, distilled vinegar, herbs, mentholated petroleum jelly, disinfectant cleaner, and even urine. These so-called cures may be worse than the disease. While some may kill fungus, they can also harm healthy skin and lead to serious complications, including infection.

Medical treatment of toenail fungus

A physician or podiatrist can diagnose a fungal infection and determine if medical treatment is warranted. Yet, medical treatment of toenail fungus is rarely quick or easy. The fact is, fungal infections are stubborn and require time, expense (especially if the treatment is not covered by your health insurance plans), and some risk. (Oral antifungals, for example, are hard on the liver.) At the same time, however, medical treatment is the best and sometimes the only way to successfully treat fungal nails.

How aggressively should a toenail fungus be treated? That determination is best made in consultation with a podiatrist, dermatologist, or medical doctor who commonly treats the condition. There a number of considerations that should factor into the decision. The appearance of the nails, while extremely embarrassing for some, is often not sufficient reason in and of itself to use expensive medications with potentially strong side effects. A fungal infection that involves more than one nail, causes pain or a secondary bacterial infection, and has been confirmed with a fungal culture is more likely to be considered a condition requiring treatment by both medical professionals and insurance providers. And as mentioned earlier, systemic medical conditions such as diabetes and circulation disorders may make it more important to treat the fungal infection aggressively with prescription medications. Conversely, because the oral medication can cause liver side effects, some people who take multiple medications for chronic conditions may not be able to take antifungal medication safely, however bad the condition of their nails. Fortunately, most people with fungal nail infections have a relatively minor infection that does not require prescription medication. They tend to do very well with nonprescription topical medications and regular nail trimming. For these people, the fungal nails are more of a nuisance than a medical condition requiring aggressive medical treatment.

4

Foot Conditions and Injuries

et's face it, the feet take a lot of abuse. They are bumped, banged, stepped on, crammed into shoes, and forced to absorb the constant pounding of thousands of daily steps. And because they support and move the body, they need, ideally, to heal quickly after they've been overused, abused, and injured. Yet today's active lifestyles provide little rest or recovery time for the feet.

Because of the constant demands on the feet, even minor foot injuries can be slow to heal. What can be done? The good news is that the body has a remarkable capacity to heal itself—under the right conditions. The conditions most important to rejuvenating and healing the feet are good pressure distribution (away from painful areas), proper cushioning and support from footwear, and, in certain cases, decreasing or changing activities until the foot improves.

A general principle to keep in mind is that the longer a foot injury has been present the longer it will take to heal. For this reason, it is important to respond to any foot injury quickly so that it can start healing immediately and you can resume normal activities as soon as possible. Also note that there are almost no treatments that will instantly resolve all pain from a foot or lower-leg injury (e.g., sprained ankle). The best long-term results tend to be achieved gradually.

Overuse and acute injuries

A large percentage of injuries to the feet are overuse injuries, meaning that they occur gradually through repetitive use. Overuse fatigues the muscles, bones, and soft tissues of our feet, making them less efficient at absorbing the forces that are transmitted from the ground up into our feet, legs, and back as we walk or run. And this, in turn, leads to stress injuries. The compounding nature of overuse becomes clear when we consider that the feet take thousands of steps each day.

Overuse injuries are deceptive. Because they occur so gradually, it is often difficult to determine their onset and cause. The gradual onset of pain also makes it easier for people to ignore overuse injuries, believing they are merely common aches and pains. And while sometimes they are, pain that lasts for more than a few days should be taken seriously.

While we are not always aware of how overuse may be injuring our feet, an acute, or sudden-onset, injury leaves no doubt about how it occurred. Ankle sprains, stubbings, or smashings (from objects falling on the feet) are some of the myriad acute foot injuries that prompt people to seek immediate treatment.

Foot injuries can be caused by seemingly trivial events as well. Occasionally, a different workout routine, a change in gait or walking pattern, or a new pair of shoes may trigger aches that persist for weeks or even months. However trivial the cause, the pain is real. It indicates the onset of an injury. And the extent of the injury is, again, compounded by the thousands of steps taken each day.

If foot pain persists for more than a day or two, there are several simple steps sufferers can do. First, make sure there is no swelling, redness, warmth, or breaks in the skin in the area of pain. If there are, seek medical attention. If these conditions are not present, limit weight-bearing activities, wear supportive shoes, and ice the painful area for twenty minutes at a time, two to three times per day. (People with circulation or sensory disorders should consult a health care provider regarding the safety of icing.) If two days of self-treatment do not improve symptoms, schedule an appointment to see a doctor, protecting the area of pain as much as possible in the meantime.

Ongoing pain, redness, swelling, warmth, and breaks in the skin indicate an acute injury and should be evaluated by a doctor as soon as possible. Delaying treatment of acute injuries can complicate them, making them worse and leading to long-term pain or even disability. Prompt professional care often makes for speedy recovery. If in doubt, err on the side of caution. Have the injury evaluated by a physician.

Factors that contribute to overuse injuries

There are many contributing factors that play a role in overuse injuries to the feet and legs. There are external factors, such as hard floors, improper footwear, weather conditions, and the demands of work (especially prolonged standing). And there are internal or personal factors, such as previous injuries, preexisting medical conditions, foot type (e.g., high arches or flat arches), footwear, medications, age, diet, and weight.

Footwear and active feet

Poor footwear can cause overuse injuries, and it can also prevent or delay the healing of injuries. Replacing footwear, then, is often an important part of not only treating injuries but also preventing future injuries. Those favorite shoes or slippers may have to be replaced with more supportive shoes or house shoes. And for people suffering from foot and lower-leg injuries, going barefoot may not be a good choice even for brief periods around the home.

Staying active is extremely important for overall health, but for those with foot or leg pain and injuries, it is equally important to rest. Temporarily decreasing, modifying, or suspending some work and fitness activities can relieve pain and aid in healing. In cases of minor pain or injury, it's okay for people to self-regulate their activity. As a general guideline, however, a doctor should be consulted if symptoms have stayed the same or worsened after one week of self-regulation.

Weight—a "big" problem

Being overweight is a key contributing factor to many types of foot and leg pain. Even a small amount of excess weight can lead to big increases in workload for the feet. Active people who are ten pounds overweight and take 10,000 steps each day, for example, subject their feet to 100,000 pounds of extra impact each day! More sedentary people who are thirty pounds overweight and take 5,000 steps per day subject their feet to 150,000 pounds of additional impact! So if good footwear, insoles, or other treatments haven't reduced or eliminated foot and leg pain, it is crucial to look at weight as the most likely culprit. The numbers are clear: losing weight reduces impact and relieves fatigue and stress.

Preexisting conditions and gait

An existing injury or medical condition can be another key risk factor for developing a foot injury. A person who has arthritis in the knee, for example, will often walk differently to minimize pain in that joint. This happens instinctively. In fact, many people who limp aren't even aware that they are doing it. When we adjust or alter our walking style, other parts of our feet and legs have to work harder, becoming more susceptible to stress and impact injuries. Treatment in such cases, then, often involves evaluating and treating the preexisting condition as well. (Note, too, that poor footwear can change a person's gait and contribute to pain and injuries.)

In order to simplify my discussion of foot conditions and injuries, I'm going to focus on three separate areas of the foot:

- heel and ankle
- midfoot (including the arches)
- forefoot (including the toes)

Of course, these areas of the feet do not function independently, so evaluating one requires understanding of the others as well.

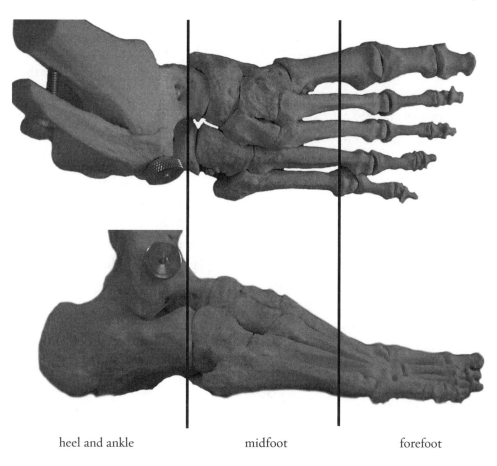

heel and ankle   midfoot   forefoot

forefoot   midfoot   heel and ankle

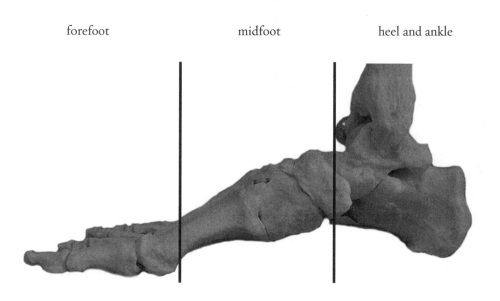

Heel and ankle conditions and injuries

The heel and ankle contain the largest bones of the foot. They play important roles when walking and running, adsorbing impact as the heel contacts the ground, then transmitting power to the forefoot to propel the body forward. Because of their importance for walking and running, the bones, tendons, and ligaments in the heel and ankle are susceptible to a number of painful conditions and potential injuries.

Plantar fasciitis and heel spurs

By far, the most common injury to the rearfoot is plantar fasciitis, or inflammation of the plantar fascia. This painful condition of the heel is also called heel spur syndrome, even though only half of those affected will develop a spur on the heel bone as a result of the condition. Plantar fasciitis is unique in that it is seen in a broad range of patients, from young marathon runners to thirty-year-old office workers to older retirees who are relatively sedentary. It seems to affect men and women equally.

The plantar fascia is a tough band of connective tissue that helps prevent the foot's arch from collapsing during standing, walking, and running. It attaches to the bottom of the heel and extends through the arch to the bases of the toes. Studies show that the plantar fascia works hardest as the heel lifts from the ground, transferring weight forward. When injured or inflamed, it hurts at the point where it attaches to the heel. The pain sometimes radiates into the arch as well.

Symptoms of plantar fasciitis include burning, tearing sensations, dull aches, or sharp, shooting pains in the heel. These symptoms are

A heel spur (shown above) develops very gradually. It is caused by long-term overuse.

especially present when rising from bed in the morning or when standing after having been sitting for a period of time. The symptoms may increase gradually over weeks or months, or they may occur suddenly after a change in activities or footwear. It is common to see this condition flare up in those who have recently started an exercise program or whose jobs require walking or standing on hard floors.

The pain associated with plantar fasciitis, strangely enough, tends to gradually diminish with walking. This is one of the unique characteristics of plantar fasciitis. There are two theories for this unusual pattern of pain. One is that the muscles on the bottom of the foot (which try to protect the injured fascia by tightening or going into a spasm) aren't able to spasm during walking activities, only after periods of rest. So part of the heel pain (in addition to that of the plantar fascia) occurs when the weight is placed on the tensed muscles. As the muscles relax, the pain decreases. The other theory is that the only time that the plantar fascia can heal itself is when no walking is occurring. So during periods of immobility—the hours of sleep, for example—the plantar fascia relaxes and shortens, relieving spasms and inflammation. Upon standing, the plantar fascia stretches, resulting in tension, inflammation, spasms, and even tearing of the fascia. The foot, basically, is reinjured each morning.

In some cases, there is no obvious cause for plantar fasciitis. In other cases, there may be many factors that contribute to it: wearing shoes that lack good arch support, being overweight, standing for long periods on hard surfaces, and exercising more than normal. Aging can be another contributing factor; the fat pad at the bottom of the heel can atrophy as we grow older. All of these conditions increase the workload placed on the plantar fascia.

Plantar fasciitis is nearing epidemic proportions in this country. A popular theory attributes the marked increase in the condition to the overuse of shoes. Proponents of this theory reason that, because we wear shoes from infancy, the muscles of the arch and other parts of the foot never develop the strength they need for a lifetime of use. As a result, the weaker muscles force the plantar fascia to work harder supporting the arch of a foot. Over time, the plantar fascia becomes inflamed, thickens, and tightens.

Treatment of plantar fasciitis

There is good news for sufferers of plantar fasciitis. Most people respond well to simple treatment options. These options can be divided into two categories: symptomatic treatment and functional treatment.

Symptomatic treatment is directed at decreasing the symptoms of plantar fasciitis—specifically, the pain and inflammation. It involves

Once you develop plantar fasciitis, you are vulnerable to recurrences. Be aware of treatments that work well for you, and use them to respond quickly at the first sign of a flare-up.

modifying activities, icing the bottom of the foot, and, if necessary, taking anti-inflammatory medication, such as ibuprofen or a cortisone injection. In minor cases that have been caught early, symptomatic treatment may completely eliminate pain. Usually, however, these measures offer only temporary relief because they do not address the underlying cause of plantar fasciitis.

Functional treatment addresses the function of the foot and the causes of the inflammation and pain of plantar fasciitis. A patient who has plantar fasciitis linked to weak arches, for example, typically benefits from the use of more supportive shoes or insoles that decrease tension of the plantar fascia. Similarly, gel heel cups commonly help those who have plantar fasciitis linked to atrophied heel fat pads.

Symptomatic treatment combined with functional treatment often yields the quickest and longest-lasting relief. The reason is simple. Combined treatment offers both prevention and management of acute flare-ups. For example, patients who ice affected feet two or three times a day and wear supportive insoles in comfortable shoes tend to remain pain-free longer and resolve the pain of flare-ups sooner than those who merely treat flare-ups with anti-inflammatory medications. Strengthening the muscles of the arch and gently stretching the foot and calf can provide better long-term results as well.

Shoes, insoles, and splints: cushioning and support

When our feet hurt, many of us intuitively seek out softer shoes or insoles. While this approach can work well for pain caused by excessive pressure, cushioning can actually make plantar fasciitis worse. The reason for this is that excessive cushioning encourages the arch of the foot to collapse, increasing stress on the planter fascia and exacerbating inflammation. So while cushioning may offer some comfort, it can work against relieving pain and inflammation. Overly soft shoes are as problematic as excessively rigid shoes.

The best footwear solutions offer a combination of cushioning and support, e.g., firm plastics or foams under the arch and denser materials in the midsole of the shoe. This combination is crucial to facilitate healing and prevent recurrences of plantar fasciitis. Investing in at least one pair of good shoes that can accommodate an insole is important for long-term pain relief.

Many people own shoes that aggravate heel pain. For example, dress shoes, high heels, and sandals often lack support and do not have room for insoles. If you have shoes that are aggravating your condition, you should either stop wearing them or at least limit their wearing time and frequency until the heel pain is resolved. If wearing a particular pair of shoes reaggravates the plantar fascia, it is best to stop wearing them entirely.

Insoles can be of great benefit for those who are already wearing supportive shoes but not experiencing relief. A cushioned heel cup or firm arch support can provide tremendous relief. Not all insoles, however, are equal. Thin, light, soft, and low-profile insoles usually offer less protection than thick, dense insoles. As with shoes, the best results are usually obtained with insoles that combine firm support with some cushioning. But even the best insoles cannot magically turn an unsupportive shoe into a supportive shoe. (If using over-the-counter insoles with good shoes has not helped, it is time to visit a podiatrist.)

Splints are another type of treatment for plantar fasciitis. They are used when sleeping or sitting. They work by keeping the foot positioned perpendicular to the leg, gently stretching the fascia and promoting its healing. Some, such as the Strassburg Sock, look like a knee-high stocking with a cord stretching from the knee to the toes. Other splints are made from lightweight padded plastic and look like walking casts. Splints often reduce the pain that

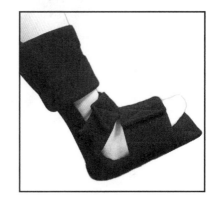

A night splint for treating plantar fasciitis. The splint keeps your foot perpendicular to your leg while you sleep.

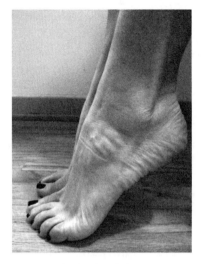

Raising the heels while seated gently stretches the plantar fascia.

comes with standing or walking after sleeping or sitting. Once you have recovered from plantar fasciitis, you no longer have to wear a splint.

Exercises for plantar fasciitis

There are some gentle stretching and strengthening exercises that may help you recover from plantar fasciitis and prevent future flare-ups. Stretching the Achilles tendon can help decrease stress and strain on the plantar fascia when walking. Two stretching exercises work well: heel lifts and calf stretches.

Heel lifts can help warm and stretch the fascia before standing. They are especially helpful for decreasing the pain when arising from bed in the morning. To stretch the fascia with heel lifts, place the feet flat on the floor from a sitting position. Then raise the heel while keeping the forefoot on the floor, thirty to fifty times for each foot. It is important to do this exercise before rising from bed in the morning or before rising from a sitting position.

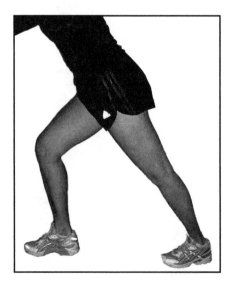
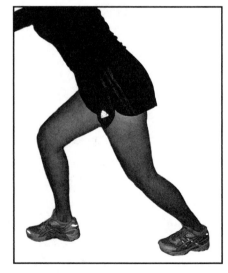

Stretching the calf muscles can help decrease tension on the plantar fascia.

To do calf stretches, lean into a wall or counter with your hands while facing forward. Extend a leg backward with your knee as straight as possible for thirty seconds and then with your knee slightly bent for thirty seconds. Concentrate on gently stretching your calf muscles. One repetition is adequate, and stretching two or three times each day is ideal. Your calf muscles will be easier and more comfortable to stretch if your plantar fascia and other muscles have first been warmed up (with heel lifts or normal walking).

To strengthen the muscles around the plantar fascia, place your feet flat on the floor from a seated position. Raise your arches while at the same time curling your toes against the floor. You can do this excercise even while wearing shoes. For more information on stretching and strengthening exercises for the ankles and feet, see Chapter 10.

Failure of plantar fasciitis treatments

While approximately 80 percent of people with plantar fasciitis can resolve their pain with conventional treatments, some may need further treatment. Cortisone injections, physical therapy, custom orthotics, shock wave treatment, and, as a last resort, surgery may be needed to resolve pain and heal the plantar fascia.

Cortisone is a powerful anti-inflammatory that can be injected into the tissue around the painful plantar fascia. Physical therapy can involve a number of treatments, include massage or soft tissue manipulation, exercise programs, and topical pain treatments. Custom orthotics are made from a cast of the feet to correct abnormal function and decrease pain on the injured area. Shock wave treatment uses pulses of sound waves generated by a powerful machine to stimulate healing of the injured plantar fascia. (This treatment is not always covered by insurance.)

Some conventional treatments may fail because conditions other than plantar fasciitis are present. Heel pain that increases or spreads over a larger area and sometimes swells despite treatment, for example, could be a sign of more serious injury, such as a bone fracture. Although uncommon, sometimes the heel bone may crack from normal walking, especially if you have osteoporosis. Some forms of arthritis can also cause heel pain that mimics plantar fasciitis.

Consult a doctor if you have heel pain that increases, spreads, or fails to respond to treatment. Only a physician can make a definitive diagnosis and recommend appropriate treatment.

Other types of heel pain

As noted above, many things besides plantar fasciitis can cause heel pain. These include rheumatoid arthritis, neuritis (inflammation of the nerves), rupture of the plantar fascia, and radiculopathy (spinal nerve root compression). However, the most common causes of pain to the back of the heel (as opposed to the bottom or side) are Achilles tendonitis, posterior heel spur, and Haglund's bumps.

Achilles tendonitis

Achilles tendonitis (inflammation of the Achilles tendon) causes pain and sometimes swelling at or just above the point where the Achilles tendon attaches to the heel bone at the back of the foot. The tendonitis usually starts without an obvious cause. Symptoms include stiffness in the back of the heel or ankle (especially in the morning) and pain or tightness when extending the leg and pulling the toes up toward the knee. In rare cases, the tendon can tear or rupture, so ongoing pain in the heel-ankle area should not be ignored.

Treatment of Achilles tendonitis can involve icing the area, taking anti-inflammatory medication, stretching the tendon gently, and wearing more supportive shoes. Wearing arch supports, heel lifts, or a splint that stretches the tendon while sleeping can sometimes help in stubborn cases. For cases that do not respond to treatment within two weeks, physicians typically order X-rays to determine if spurring, or calcification of the tendon, is present.

Posterior heel spurs

Posterior heel spurs (calcification of the Achilles tendon) cause pain to the back of the heel either at the heel bone or up the tendon above the heel. Calcification causes the Achilles tendon and soft tissue around the bone to lose elasticity, which leads to inflammation, pain, and swelling. This condition can only be diagnosed after taking an

X-ray of the heel. Pressure from shoes and activity usually make symptoms worse. For some, even the pressure against the heels when sleeping can cause pain.

Treatment for posterior heel spurs can be difficult and should be done under the direction of a physician. Treatment usually involves physical therapy, oral anti-inflammatory medication, icing, stretching, and shoe changes. Some people find that their symptoms can be improved by wearing shoes that have an open back, such as clogs or sandals. Padding (such as moleskin) can be added to the heel cup of the shoe to decrease pressure on the painful area. A gel heel sleeve is commercially available for padding the painful area when wearing shoes or sleeping, as is a larger, softer pad made just for use in bed. (These larger, softer pads work well for Haglund's bumps, too.)

Haglund's bumps

Haglund's bumps are painful but benign enlargements of the heel bone. They are often clearly visible or easily felt. Developing very slowly over the course of years, the enlargements are caused by the continuous tension of an overly tight Achilles tendon or pressure from footwear.

Haglund's bumps become painful when irritated by shoes. In some cases, an inflamed bursa (fluid pocket) will develop at the site. In these instances, the bump appears red and swollen and is very tender to the touch. It is common for Haglund's bumps to form on each heel; although they don't always hurt equally, or even at all. Though benign, the bumps can continue to increase in size over time. As they enlarge, they can become an increasingly painful problem.

Haglund's bumps do not go away or shrink unless surgically removed. Fortunately, very few people have to resort to surgery; most people can manage the symptoms with conservative methods. Treatment can be as simple as adding a horseshoe-shaped pad to the heel cup of the shoe to decrease pressure. A gel heel sleeve can work well, too. In more stubborn cases, a shoe repair shop or certified pedorthist can permanently modify the heel of the shoe to decrease pressure on the bump. For those who cannot tolerate any pressure on the heel from shoes but do not want to resort to surgery, wearing open-back shoes, such as clogs or sandals, is often a satisfactory solution.

Ankle pain and injuries

By far, the most common injury to the ankle is an ankle sprain. An ankle sprain is usually very obvious when it occurs—a sudden twisting of the ankle results in pain and swelling. Repeated or severe ankle sprains can predispose a person to chronic ankle pain that surfaces years or even decades after the the original injury. Other types of ankle injuries are not as easily identified and often occur so gradually that no single cause is apparent.

Ankle sprains

The most common cause of acute pain in the ankle and one of the most undertreated injuries is an ankle sprain. Ankle sprains are, of course, common in athletics, but they also occur during normal walking. Walking on uneven or slippery surfaces, wearing high-heeled shoes, having poor balance, walking on stairs, and having "weak" ankles from previous injuries are all common causes of ankle sprains.

Ankle sprains usually occur when the ankle rolls outward during a step or fall, wrenching or twisting ligaments of the ankle and rupturing blood vessels. Pain and swelling may be immediate and, in more severe sprains, a lot of bruising occurs as well. Of special concern are sounds or sensations of popping, snapping, or tearing at the time of the injury. These are indicators that a more serious injury may have occurred, including a ruptured ligament or a broken bone. Both acute and chronic (recurring) sprains should be evaluated by a medical professional.

Treatment of sprains varies, but most commonly, some combination of rest, ice, compression, and elevation is used. This combination of treatments is often referred to by the acronym R.I.C.E.

- **Rest**: Get off your feet as soon as possible.
- **Ice**: Apply ice frequently but not more than twenty minutes at a time (to avoid frostbite).
- **Compression**: Wrap an elastic bandage around your ankle.
- **Elevation**: Raise your ankle.

Applying the R.I.C.E method as soon as possible will help to minimize swelling. Aspirin, acetaminophen, or ibuprofen can also be taken to relieve pain.

The first 24 to 48 hours following an ankle sprain are the most important and can provide clues about the severity of the injury. Minor sprains do not bruise, swell very little if at all, and allow walking with no or minimal pain. These sprains usually heal quickly (within a few days) and without complications. Moderate to severe sprains cause bruising, swelling, and hurt when weight is placed on the foot. Symptoms persist for days, weeks, or even months if not treated properly. These types of sprains can involve tearing (rupture) of ligaments or tendons and sometimes injuries to bones or cartilage. Moderate to severe sprains should be seen by a medical professional. Neglected or untreated ankle sprains can lead to chronic pain, instability of the ankle, and arthritis.

An often overlooked aspect of even minor ankle sprains is the damage done to the nerves around the ankle. We all have system of nerves that we use for movement and balance. These nerves are called proprioceptors. If you close your eyes and point your index finger in different directions, it is your proprioceptors that tell you which direction your finger is pointing. The proprioceptors of the ankle are often injured when the ankle is sprained. This is why people often feel like they can't "trust their ankle" to support their weight. Because their proprioceptive nerve fibers aren't transmitting orienting signals properly, the ankle feels unstable. This lack of stability is especially apparent when walking on uneven surfaces. Special exercises and balancing movements can help to rehabilitate injured proprioceptive nerves.

For some ankle sprains, additional treatment may be needed. Those vulnerable to repeated ankle sprains may need physical therapy and changes in shoes to strengthen the ankles and regain stability. Firm shoes that keep the feet close to the ground will provide a more stable platform than cushioned shoes that elevate the feet.

"Fallen arches" (posterior tibial tendon dysfunction)

Ankle pain that is located only on the inside of the ankle (the side closer to the other foot) is usually a sign of a condition called posterior tibial tendon dysfunction, or PTTD. (The posterior tibial tendon stretches from the lower leg to the arch of the foot and is part of the main structure that supports the arch.) Those with flat feet or

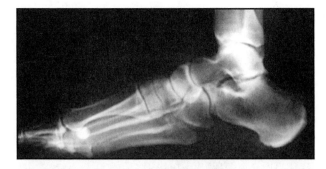

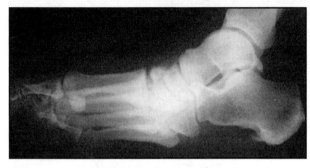

The X-rays above show a foot with healthy midfoot joints and normal arch height (top) and a foot with collapsing midfoot joints and arthritis (bottom). Note how the midfoot "sags" in the lower X-ray.

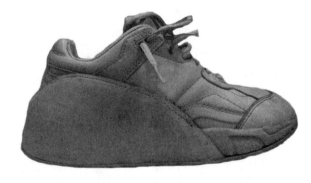

This shoe has been customized with an aggressive external arch support to treat posterior tibial tendon dysfunction.

feet that have arches that collapse excessively are most vulnerable to this injury, which is why the condition is sometimes referred to as fallen arches. The collapsing arch excessively strains the posterior tibial tendon on every step. Over the course of years, this strain can cause the tendon to become inflamed and then to stretch and tear.

Flat-footed women between the ages of forty and sixty and overweight individuals seem to be most affected by PTTD.

The pain associated with posterior tibial tendon dysfunction often extends from behind the ankle bone into the arch of the foot. There is a simple self-test to determine if the posterior tibial tendon is injured. If you feel pain or an increase in pain when shifting your weight to the affected foot and rising up onto your toes, then it is likely that the tendon is injured. If treated early, the tendon usually heals. In severe cases or, if left untreated, the tendon can stretch and, ultimately, tear.

Treatment of PTTD starts with a visit to a podiatrist or

orthopedist. He or she will determine the extent of the injury and assess the best ways to support the arch and heel—the key to treating the disorder. The mildest cases of this injury tend to respond to simple shoe changes and over-the-counter insoles. Other cases, however, require treatment with rigid shoes, custom orthotics, or braces.

Osteoarthritis in the ankle

There are numerous types of arthritis, but a common type in weight-bearing joints is called osteoarthritis. Osteoarthritis is caused by either a traumatic injury to the joint, such as a fracture that breaks a bone in or near the joint, or slow deterioration of the cartilage inside the joint.

Like any weight-bearing joint, the ankle joint is susceptible to osteoarthritis. The cartilage in the ankle joint can break down over time on its own. A preexisting injury at or near the ankle joint can also lead to arthritis. It is not unusual for arthritis to develop in an ankle joint years after a fracture or other serious injury. Arthritis in the ankle joint can be especially disabling because the ankle is a large joint responsible for a broad range of motion.

There is no cure for any type of arthritis. Treatment is directed at controlling arthritic pain, reducing inflammation, and decreasing the workload on the joints. For those with osteoarthritis, this treatment can include anti-inflammatory medications, changes in shoes, or the use of orthotics or braces.

Midfoot injuries and conditions

The heel and ankle are connected to the forefoot and toes by a number of small bones and joints in the middle portion of the foot, called the midfoot. The structures of the midfoot, including a number of small joints, help transfer weight from the heel to the toes during walking and running. Even normal walking and running require a tremendous amount of work from these midfoot joints. It is not surprising, then, that these small joints can become arthritic.

Arthritis of the midfoot

The most common cause of midfoot arthritis is a flat or unstable foot, which causes the midfoot joints to work even harder than normal. Over the course of years, the cartilage that protects these joints starts to break down, increasing friction at the joints. The greater the deterioration of the cartilage, the more pronounced the symptoms. Symptoms of midfoot arthritis include achiness, pain, bone spurs (bony bumps) on the top of the foot, and, sometimes, grinding sensations in the affected joint or joints. X-rays of an arthritic midfoot will, as you might expect, show irregular joint space, bone spurs, and signs of bone stress.

If a flat foot or collapsing arch is a contributing factor to midfoot arthritis, then an important part of treatment is supporting the arch with an insole or orthotics and rigid shoes. By supporting the arch, the flattening of the midfoot is controlled, reducing the stress on the arthritic joints. Arthritis caused by previous injuries such as fractures or severe sprains are treated similarly.

Arch pain (plantar fibroma)

A benign tumor of soft, fibrous tissue—called a plantar fibroma—can form on the arch of the foot. The cause of this growth is not known. The fibroma usually grows very slowly and sometimes disappears without any treatment. It can be as small as a pea or a few inches in diameter. It usually only hurts during weight-bearing activities. If a plantar fibroma is persistently painful, it can be satisfactorily treated with custom-molded orthotics that decrease pressure at the site. Occasionally injection therapy or topical treatments can relieve symptoms. In rare instances, the fibroma must be removed surgically.

Extensor tendonitis

Extensor tendonitis is an inflammation of the tendons on the top of the midfoot. Extensor tendonitis can be caused by tight or tightly laced shoes, bony bumps on the top of the foot (which aggravate the tendons), or a tight Achilles tendon. Successful treatment usually requires only icing the site, taking anti-inflammatory medication, and performing gentle foot-stretching exercises. If a pair of shoes is the cause of the tendonitis, they should be exchanged for better fitting shoes. Stubborn cases may need physical therapy under a physician's supervision.

Distal plantar fasciitis

Plantar fasciitis doesn't always cause pain to the bottom of the heel. Sometimes, the pain is located in the arch of the foot. As with non-distal plantar fasciitis, pain is typically felt in the morning after arising from bed or after standing and improves after a few minutes of walking. Often, the pain is worsened by pulling the toes up and pushing on a tight cord of tissue that can be felt on the bottom of the arch. Treatment for distal plantar fasciitis is the same as for regular plantar fasciitis. (See p. 64.)

Forefoot injuries and conditions

Injuries to the forefoot are often caused by a combination of changes in the alignment of the toes and an uneven distribution of pressure at the ball of the foot. People often mistakenly assume that only the heel is impacted when we step, but the force of impact on the forefoot as the body is pushed forward can be just as intense, or even more so. Repeated thousands of times each day, step impact on the forefoot can take a toll. (Hammertoes and bunions, the most common sources of forefoot pain, are discussed in Chapter 5.)

Stress fractures—the "sneaky" injury

A stress fracture is a small crack in a bone. Most people who are diagnosed with stress fractures in the forefoot or elsewhere are surprised that they have a broken bone. The reason for their surprise is that they do not recall doing anything that may have broken the bone, such as falling or being stepped on. In most cases, they were simply going about their normal routine and suddenly began to notice

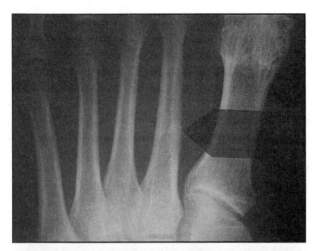

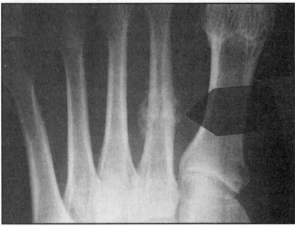

Top: One week after a patient began to experience pain and swelling in the forefoot. The hairline crack in the bone is barely visible next to the arrow.

Bottom: The same patient four weeks later. The cloudy bone callus indicates that the fracture is healing.

pain. Others can develop stress fractures after increasing activity, changing shoes, or as a consequence of weakened bones. In fact, stress fractures can be the first symptom of osteopenia or osteoporosis, medical conditions involving the loss of bone mass and density.

Stress fractures differ from acute fractures in that they don't occur suddenly. They develop very slowly— sometimes over weeks or even months. What often starts as an ache during walking can gradually develop into throbbing pain and swelling. Some stress fractures do not swell or cause enough pain to stop a person from walking, and for this reason, it is easy for many people to dismiss the pain, thinking it a minor ache or pain that will go away. Meanwhile, the small crack in the bone can "spider," or advance, much as a cracked windshield does if not repaired.

Untreated stress fractures can progress from a tiny crack to a complete break of the bone. For this reason, as well as the potential for osteoporosis, it is important to seek medical treatment for persistent pain.

Stress fractures in the foot are most common in the forefoot's metatarsal bones. They occur less commonly in the bones of the midfoot, heel, and lower leg. The metatarsals are vulnerable to injury because they are long, thin bones that are under tremendous strain on every step. Because it is the longest, the second metatarsal, which leads to the second toe (next to the big toe), is the metatarsal injured most often. Pain that occurs when pushing directly on the bone or when hopping on one foot usually indicates a metatarsal fracture.

In the first few weeks of injury, stress fractures can easily be misdiagnosed because they are usually imperceptibly small. So small, in fact, that they are not visible on X-rays. Later, X-rays will often show a bump on the bone in the area of pain. The bump is called a bone callus and is a sign of a healing stress fracture. The bone callus, however, can take three to four weeks to become evident on an X-ray.

If there is pain when pressing on the bone and swelling is present but the X-ray fails to show a crack, your doctor may decide to treat it as a fracture under the assumption that the fracture just isn't visible. There is also a condition called a stress reaction, where the bone has not cracked yet but will if not protected adequately.

Most stress fractures are treated with doctor-prescribed fracture boots or stiff shoes worn from four to eight weeks. The idea is to immobilize the foot, relieving stress on the fractured bone and promoting healing. Walking in the boot or shoe is acceptable as long as it does not cause pain. For those whose jobs involve long periods of walking or standing, a temporary change in work routine may be necessary. Crutches or wheelchairs are almost never needed unless the heel bone is involved or there are fractures of multiple bones. If a doctor suspects that osteoporosis is present, he or she may recommend a bone density test. If osteoporosis is found, additional treatment will most likely be needed.

Pain in the forefoot bones (metatarsalgia)

Metatarsalgia literally means "achy metatarsal," and the condition is simply a sore bone or bones in the forefoot. Forefoot stress fractures are often misdiagnosed as metatarsalgia because the initial symptoms—aches in a bone or bones—are so similar. It is important that physicians differentiate metatarsalgia from a metatarsal stress fracture to ensure proper treatment for both conditions. If you are experiencing pain in your forefoot, ask your doctors to consider both as possible causes of your pain. Even for experienced medical professionals, it is not always easy to differentiate between metatarsalgia and a stress fracture.

Metatarsalgia is usually easily treated, responding well to wearing more supportive shoes (women should avoid high-heeled shoes) and adding a metatarsal pad to the shoe. A metatarsal pad is a teardrop-shaped pad that helps distribute pressure evenly over the forefoot. It can be directly added to a shoe or insole—a removable insole, ideally, so that the pad and insole can be used in more than one pair of shoes.

The best metatarsal pads are made from wool felt. They usually require the expertise of a podiatrist for correct placement. Placing the pads too far toward the toes, for example, increases metatarsal pain instead of relieving it. Thin foam or gel metatarsal pads are less durable, more difficult to place, and often take several days to become comfortable. Talk to a podiatrist about what type of metatarsal pad would be best for you to use.

Some shoes or insoles have built-in metatarsal arch support, or metatarsal "button." Tacco insoles, Birkenstock, and Finn Comfort shoes and sandals have a small support at the end of the arch, which can be of benefit to those with forefoot pain. These supports, however, are minimal and may not relieve pain for everyone. A podiatrist can help determine if shoes or insoles with metatarsal arch support would be beneficial.

Pain in the base of the toes (capsulitis)

A type of metatarsalgia that affects the ends of the metatarsals at the ball of the foot is called capsulitis. It is an inflammation of the soft tissue, or capsule, that surrounds the joint where the metatarsal joins with the small bones leading to the toe. This condition is often caused by hammertoes, which increase pressure on the capsule. A callus on the bottom of the foot in the area of pain also is commonly seen with capsulitis, especially when it affects the metatarsal joint of the second toe (the toe next to the big toe).

Capsulitis is treated by relieving the pressure on the painful capsule. This is done with an insole or orthotics that may need to be modified with a metatarsal pad. The addition of a metatarsal pad to existing shoes without an insole may work for some. Gel forefoot sleeves offer a third way to treat capsulitis. The sleeves are sometimes more bulky than thin insoles or metatarsal pads, but they work well, especially if the plantar fat pad on the bottom of the forefoot has shrunk.

Pain under the big toe joint (sesamoiditis)

There are two small bones located under the ball of the foot at the bottom of the big toe joint. These two bones are called sesamoids, ostensibly because they resemble sesame seeds. The sesamoids are embedded in tendons and are part of a pulley system that allows them to glide under the big toe joint as weight is transferred during walking. This helps to stabilize the big toe joint. Occasionally, the sesamoids become tender or painful and can even fracture. X-rays are necessary for accurate diagnosis.

Treatment of sesamoiditis often consists of attempting to distribute pressure away from the site with a modified insole. Icing the area and taking anti-inflammatory medications are other common treatments. Metatarsal pads, arch supports, and a special forefoot modification to the insole called a reverse Morton's extension can be used to protect the painful area. Wearing shoes with good cushioning (but not too much cushioning) and avoiding shoes with elevated heels are important to healing until pain subsides. A gel forefoot sleeve can work well for this condition as well.

Pain in the big toe joint

People sometimes assume that a painful big toe joint means gout, but bunions and arthritic changes are more common causes of pain in the big toe joint. In fact, I've had many a patient present to my office complaining of gout, only to find, after an exam and X-rays, that they actually have a bunion or an arthritic condition called hallux limitus (also known as hallux rigidus). All three conditions are characterized by redness, pain, and swelling, which can make it difficult to distinguish between them. But while gout is less common than the other conditions, it is often much more painful

Bunions and hallux limitus are discussed in Chapter 5. Gout is a condition caused by the build-up of uric acid crystals in the bloodstream. The uric acid crystals look like shards of glass when viewed under a microscope. Certain foods can trigger an attack of gout by raising the level of uric acid in the blood. Seafood, nuts, red meat, and beer or wine can elevate uric levels. High levels of uric acid in the blood stream crystallize and deposit in joints when exposed to cooler temperatures. Since the feet are often the coolest parts of the body, gout attacks are most common in the feet.

Those who have experienced attacks of gout describe pain, redness, and swelling at the joint. Many complain of a pain so intense that even the light touch of a breeze or bedsheet is excruciating. Treatment must be initiated by a doctor, and it usually involves taking anti-inflammatory medication and avoiding the foods that triggered the attack. A doctor may prescribe additional medications to control chronic attacks.

Toe fractures

Fractures of the toes often occur by bumping into a piece of furniture or dropping something on the foot. They are probably the most neglected fracture because many people are convinced that nothing can be done for toe fractures. While it is true that wearing loose shoes and taping the injured toe to an adjacent toe is often all that is needed for treatment, some toe fractures can be significant enough to warrant additional medical treatment for proper healing and to minimize the risk of long-term complications.

Fractures to the big toe, for example, should be treated by a doctor. Likewise, toes that are bent following a suspected break or dislocation should be seen immediately. Toes that don't improve quickly with self-care should also be looked at by a doctor. In these cases, the break may have to be set for the bone to heal properly.

A warning: Popular wisdom has it that if you can move the injured area, then it is not broken. This is simply not true. Most fractured bones or joints are capable of moving. Note, too, that bruising, swelling, and redness will be present for most injuries to the toes whether that injury is a contusion, dislocation, or fracture.

Arthritic conditions of the forefoot

Pain in one or more of the joints in the ball of the foot may be a symptom of arthritis. In addition to pain, symptoms of arthritis include stiffness, swelling, and redness localized to the ball of the foot or bases of the toes. There are different types of arthritis, and sometimes it can be difficult to diagnose the exact source of the symptoms. Some arthritic conditions are caused by autoimmune or metabolic disorders, while others are caused by obesity or previous trauma. There is no cure for any type of arthritis. Treatments are aimed at protecting the joints and addressing the symptoms with anti-inflammatory medications. The most common types of arthritis in the ball of the foot are rheumatoid arthritis and osteoarthritis.

Rheumatoid arthritis affects multiple joints simultaneously. An early symptom of the condition is stiffness in the hands, especially in the morning. Fever, fatigue, and malaise can occur as well. The first symptoms of rheumatoid arthritis are rarely felt in the feet, but the feet joints do become affected over time. As rheumatoid arthritis progresses, the joints at the ball of the foot may enlarge and the toes lose their normal alignment. In severe cases, nodules can form around the joints as well. These nodules can become painful from the pressure of walking or wearing shoes. This condition should be managed by your primary care doctor or rheumatologist. Podiatrists often prescibe custom orthotics to decrease pressure on painful joints, and surgery may be appropriate for severe cases.

Unlike rheumatoid arthritis, which affects multiple joints, osteoarthrities can affect just one joint or a couple of adjacent joints. While osteoarthritis in the midfoot (discussed earlier) can occur with or without trauma, osteoarthritis of the forefoot joints is usually the result of a previous injury, such as a forefoot fracture or severe sprain.

The injury causes a gradual deterioration of the cartilage, the symptoms of which can take years or even decades to make themselves felt. As with any arthritic condition, X-rays are needed to diagnose osteoarthritis. Treatment is directed at protecting the joint with orthotics and proper footwear and using anti-inflammatory medications as needed. Surgery is an option in severe cases.

Morton's neuroma

Burning pain or numbness in the toes may be caused by a condition called Morton's neuroma. It is most common between the third and fourth toes. Morton's neuroma is the result of an enlarged and inflamed nerve in the forefoot. Symptoms are usually triggered by long periods of walking and standing. They may worsen during certain activities or while wearing certain shoes. Morton's neuroma seems to be more common in those with wide feet and who wear shoes that are too narrow, and may be the result of tight shoes squeezing the feet together, causing mechanical irritation to the nerve.

Relief can sometimes be achieved by removing the shoe and rubbing the painful area. But more commonly, treatment consists of anti-inflammatory therapy, footwear changes, insole modifications (like metatarsal pads), and, occasionally, cortisone injections or surgery to decompress or remove the nerve.

There are other common conditions affecting the toes and toe joints in addition to the few mentioned here. In fact, two of these conditions—hammertoes and bunions—are so common and have so much *in* common, they merit their own separate chapter.

5

Hammertoes and Bunions

Most of us can expect to see changes in our toes as we age. As the soft tissue in the foot shrinks and the skin atrophies with age, bones can become more prominent, increasing the risk of the foot rubbing against the inside of the shoe and forming painful calluses. These changes can result in two common toe conditions: hammertoes and bunions. A third condition, called hallux limitus, an arthritic condition of the great toe joint, is also relatively common and is discussed at the end of this chapter.

Both hammertoes and bunions start out as muscle imbalances in the feet that the bones and joints try to adapt to and compensate for. Sometimes these imbalances are caused by genetic or hereditary factors. But other factors, such as arthritis, injury, and footwear, can also contribute to hammertoes and bunions. In fact, people who go barefoot or wear sandals a lot are less likely than others to develop hammertoes or bunions. So it is clear that shoes are probably the most significant contributing factor to these conditions.

Hammertoes and bunions are not reversible. Changing shoes, wearing insoles or orthotics, or using

Hammertoes and bunions do not develop overnight. Patients come to me convinced that new shoes, insoles, or physical activities have suddenly caused hammertoes or bunions to form. This is highly unlikely. New shoes can make hammertoes more painful, but the condition takes a long time to develop. Only an acute trauma, such as a fracture, can cause an instantly noticeable bunion or hammertoe, but even this is extremely unusual.

83

splints may relieve the pain of these conditions, especially pain caused by rubbing, but none of these treatments will correct a hammertoe or remove a bunion. The only way to correct a hammertoe or remove a bunion is surgery. However, surgical correction is a last resort. The first step is to attempt to manage the discomfort with the treatments described below.

Hammertoes

A hammertoe is a contracted, or permanently bent, toe that can cause pain in the toe or forefoot. The muscles that control the toe need to be in perfect balance to keep the toe in its naturally straight position. But biomechanical changes in toe muscles and years of confining footwear can force a toe to bend. Over time, the toe remains in this unnatural position. Hammertoes are most common in the smaller toes and rarely affect the big toe. In some cases, only the second toe is affected; in others, all of the small toes are contracted or bent. In the most severe cases, a hammertoe actually starts to cross over the toe next to it.

The fourth and fifth toes, or two smallest toes, often contract in a different way from the second and third toes. These "outside" toes not only bend, but also rotate under slightly so that a person is practically walking on the sides of the toes. This rotation happens because the muscles of the fourth and fifth toes align differently from the other toes and because the narrow toe box of many shoes tends to squeeze and roll these toes under toward the big toe.

A hammertoe can cause pain in a number of ways. As the toe contracts, the joint in the middle of the toe is pushed upward and is then subjected to pressure from the shoes. This results in the development of painful

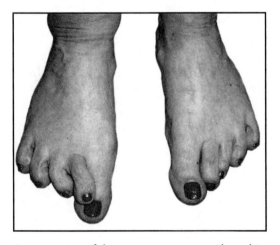

Contractures of the toes are pronounced on this patient's right foot, and the second toe has crossed over the big toe. The toes on her left foot are relatively straight.

red, irritated, blistered skin and, over time, a callus. A painful callus can also form on the end of the toe from rubbing against the bottom of the shoe. Hammertoes with rotation can add to the pain, as occasionally a very painful callus, or corn, forms between the rolled toes. Pain on the side of the toe from pressure against the ground or shoe can develop as well. There are also two unique types of calluses associated with rotated hammertoes: pinch calluses and Lister's corns. Pinch calluses form in a ridge under the toe resulting from the "pinching" of the toe between the adjacent toe and the ground. A Lister's corn can form next to the outside border of the toenail, again from pressure. These types of calluses can be especially painful.

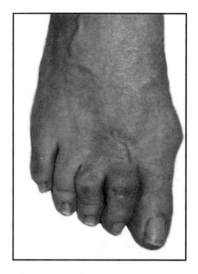

This patient has hammertoes in the second and third digits of her foot.

Hammertoes can be flexible or rigid. A hammertoe is considered flexible if the affected toe can be straightened with the fingers. If the toe cannot be straightened with the fingers, then it is considered rigid. Flexibility and rigidity determine to some degree the course of treatment to follow. Flexible hammertoes tend to respond better than rigid hammertoes to nonsurgical treatments. Conversely, rigid hammertoes often require surgical treatment.

Other problems related to hammertoes

Hammertoes can change how the forefoot distributes pressure. As a hammertoe becomes progressively more bent, the pressure on the joint between the toe and the ball of the foot increases. Eventually, this increased pressure can cause inflammation in the joint, a condition called capsulitis. This condition must be treated in addition to treating the hammertoe. Treatment for capsulitis usually involves the use of insoles, metatarsal pads, or orthotics.

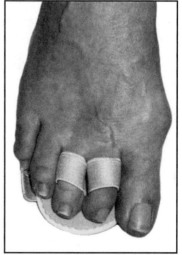

An elastic hammertoes splint helps straighten the toes.

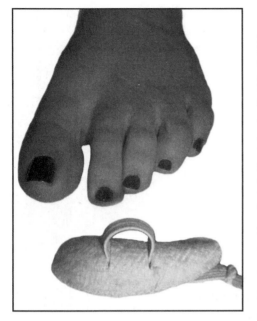

Hammertoes can create additional problems. When the toes contract, the large, protective pad on the bottom of the forefoot, called the plantar fat pad, can be affected. This pad protects and cushions the bones at the ball of the foot. As the hammertoes contract, the fat pad is pushed away from the bones, and the bones are no longer protected from the impact of walking and running. For some, the pain from the displaced fat pad is much worse than the pain from the hammertoes themselves. Padded forefoot sleeves, insoles or orthotics with a metatarsal pad, and cushioning for the forefoot all work well to treat this condition.

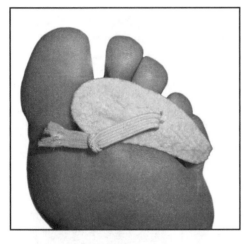

This hammertoe splint loops over a single toe and decreases contracture by filling in the space under the toes.

Treatment of hammertoes

Treating hammertoes involves either alleviating the pressure on painful areas from pressure, splinting the toes to decrease the contracture, or both. As mentioned above, flexible hammertoes are usually easier to treat; rigid, overlapping, or rotating hammertoes tend to be more resistant to conservative treatment. Keep in mind that no treatment works the same for everybody. If you have a problem with hammertoes, you will need to use trial and error to find the treatments and products that work best for you. Often, the best solutions involve combining treatments and individualizing them to meet particular needs in particular situations.

The first step in treating hammertoes is to avoid shoes that put pressure on your toes. For some people, this may mean wearing shoes with additional depth in the toe box. Proper shoes are especially important for work and fitness activities, when the demands on the feet are the greatest.

In addition to wearing better shoes, you can pad and splint the toes to protect the painful areas. Gel toe sleeves slip over the toe like a sock to provide padding. A hammertoe splint loops over the toe, pulling it into a straighter position. Combining the gel toe sleeve with the splint works well for some people. "Corn pads" are foam pads with adhesive backing that are applied to the painful area. This is a good option if you wear shoes that do not accommodate other pads or splints. Avoid medicated corn pads. They contain acid that can burn or injure the skin.

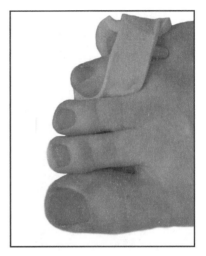

A hammertoe splint for the fourth and fifth toes.

Metatarsal pads placed in the shoe to relieve pressure can help if the hammertoes are contributing to pain at the ball of the foot.

Painful hammertoes that do not improve with conservative treatment may warrant surgical correction.

Bunions

Bunions are one of the most common complaints that podiatrists hear from their patients. A history of bunions tend to run in families. They are also more common among women than men, but this may be because women's shoes are, on the whole, more constricting and deforming than men's shoes.

A bunion is a somewhat complex change in the joint of the big toe in which a bony enlargement develops at the base of the toe, forcing it to angle toward the second toe. A bunion can involve one or both joints of the big toe. It is a progressive deformity that will continue to distort the angle of the toe joint. Pain results from the foot swelling and rubbing

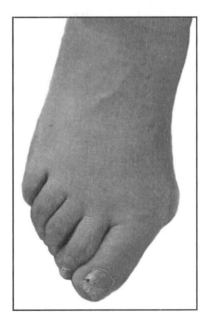

A bunion. Note the enlarged joint at the base of the big toe and the angle of the big toe as it bends toward the smaller toes.

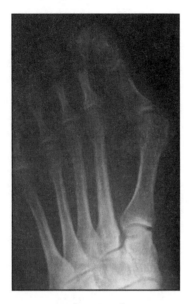

An X-ray of a severe bunion. The big toe has started to cross over the second toe.

against the inside of the shoe. Bunions can also contribute to the development of arthritis in the joint, which also causes pain.

Bunions are caused by a combination of structural vulnerability of the toe joint and poor footwear. No one is born with a bunion, but certain foot types are more vulnerable than others to the formation of a bunion. A big toe joint that is too flexible, an arch that collapses too easily, or a joint surface with a particular contour (something that can only be seen using an X-ray) are structural vulnerabilities that contribute to the formation of a bunion. Combine these structural vulnerabilities with improperly fitted footwear, and a bunion is quite often the result.

If you have a bunion, your initial treatment will involve changes in footwear: wearing wider shoes, using a supportive insole or orthotics, or inserting a toe spacer between the big toe and second toe. For large bunions, shoes may have to be stretched or cut to decrease the pressure on the bunion. If adjustments to footwear fail to solve the problem, then surgical options may be considered. A number of surgical procedures are available, depending on the size of the bunion, the level of pain, and the lifestyle of the patient.

Nonsurgical treatment of bunions

Improving the alignment of the joint and alleviating pressure on the bunion are the keys to decreasing pain and discomfort. Try these conservative treatment options before considering surgery.

Shoes

Sometimes, female patients have a hard time giving up wearing narrow, pointed shoes because they want to be fashionable. But being fashionable should not be a justification for deforming your feet. It is absolutely imperative that you wear foot-healthy shoes if you have a bunion. Shoes that have appropriate forefoot width and a round toe box will not squeeze the toes into unnatural positions. To decrease pressure on the bunion and reduce inflammation and swelling, you must wear a shoe with sufficient width for the forefoot and a rounded rather than pointed toe box. In many cases, a pedorthist or skilled shoe repair shop can modify shoes by stretching them or sewing in panels of upper material to widen shoes to accommodate the bunion and relieve pain.

Toe spacers

A toe spacer helps maintain the normal alignment of the big toe joint by pushing the big toe away from the second toe. This, in turn, helps to relieve pressure on the joint. Toe spacers are made from foam, rubber, or silicone gel and are available in different sizes. As with many of the products mentioned in this book, it may take some trial and error to determine the most effective spacer for your foot.

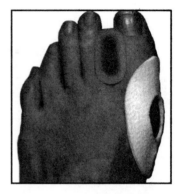

A bunion shield cushions the bunion with padding. In this picture, a toe spacer is used between the big toe and second toe as well, to improve alignment and relieve pain.

Bunion shields (padding)

Bunion shields can be made from moleskin, rubber, or silicone gel and are found at most pharmacies. They are worn inside the shoe. Some adhere to the skin while others loop over the big toe and protect the bunion with a cup-shaped pad. As their name suggests, bunion shields prevent pressure on the bunion.

Bunion splints

Bunion splints are worn when shoes are not being worn. They cannot reverse or heal a bunion, but some people do experience pain relief when wearing them. Bunion splints straighten the affected toe. There are a number of different styles of bunion splints. Some are made of padded fabric and secured with Velcro straps.

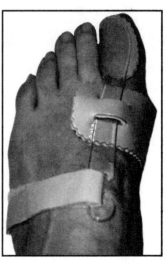

A bunion splint.

Insoles and orthotics

Insoles and orthotics can help decrease pressure on the big toe joint by supporting the foot and controlling some of the forces that caused the bunion to develop in the first place. When combined with a toe spacer, insoles and orthotics are especially effective.

Surgical correction of bunions

Bunions that have not improved with basic treatment may need to be treated surgically. There are numerous surgical procedures, and a

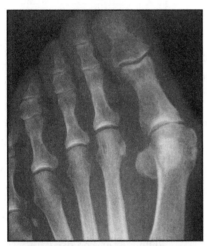

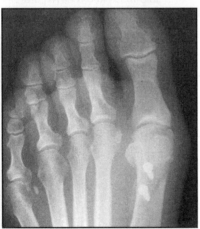

podiatrist or orthopedist can recommend a procedure that is right for you. Fortunately, many of the procedures allow for a relatively quick recovery. In fact, some procedures will have the patient walking in a protective cast the day of surgery and returning to regular shoes in three to five weeks. The most severe bunions, however, may require more complex surgical procedures, after which a patient may have to wear a cast and use crutches for up to six weeks.

Simple bunion surgery involves removing the bump of bone and releasing contracted tissues. More involved procedures require cutting the metatarsal bone, straightening it, and then fastening the bone fragments together with screws or wires until they heal. Sometimes, it is necessary to fuse a joint in the midfoot to correct a stubborn bunion. This means putting screws through the joint at the base of the first metatarsal to eliminate the instability that is causing the bunions to form.

Studies have shown that patient satisfaction with bunion surgery is approximately 90

X-rays of a bunion before surgery (top) and after surgery (bottom) with screws holding bone in correct position.

percent. However, there is always the possibility of complications. These potential complications include joint stiffness, infection, painful scarring, unresolved pain, recurrence of the bunion, the failure of the bone to heal, and chronic swelling in the foot.

Bunions can recur after surgery. The surgery will remove the bunion, but if the conditions that produced it are still present (e.g., poor footwear), a new bunion will form. Wearing supportive shoes is especially important after bunion surgery.

Other types of bunions

Although less common than bunions and hammertoes, two other conditions—tailor's bunions and hallux limitus—can also make walking and wearing shoes very painful.

Tailor's bunions

Tailor's bunions, also called "bunionettes," are small bumps on the forefoot at the base of the little toe. While much less common than bunions of the big toe joint, both types of bunions are cause by the same thing: pressure. Tailor's bunions are so named because they were once commonly seen in tailors, who tended to sit crosslegged on the floor. Long hours of pressing their feet against the floor this way caused pain and enlargement of the little toe joint. Tailor's bunions tend to become red and painful when aggravated by pressure from tight shoes. They are more common in people who have wide feet and are therefore more likely to feel pressure when wearing shoes.

There are not as many treatment options for Tailor's bunions as there are for bunions of the big toe. Treatments include stretching or padding the shoes and surgically removing the bunions. Surgical correction for tailor's bunions is much less involved than that for bunions of the big toe, so recovery is often quicker and easier, with less risk of complications.

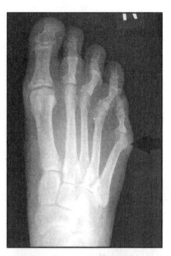

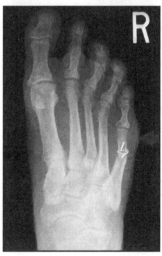

A tailor's bunion before (top) and after (bottom) surgical correction.

Hallux limitus—arthritis of the big toe joint

Hallux limitus or hallux rigidus (meaning, literally, limited big toe or rigid big toe) is a common arthritic condition at the base of the big toe. The condition is also sometimes called a "dorsal bunion" because, instead of producing a bony prominence on the side of the joint like a conventional bunion, the bump forms on the top (or dorsal aspect) of the joint. Hallux limitus can be caused by an old injury, gradual wear and tear over time, or a combination of both. The bony bump that forms on the joint will progressively enlarge and may become increasingly painful as it rubs against a shoe. Like other forms of arthritis, there is stiffness and soreness in the joint. X-rays are necessary to diagnose this condition.

Treatment for hallux limitus typically involves supporting the foot and decreasing the workload on the joint. Less severe cases may respond well to orthotics and shoe changes. Supporting the arch with a firm insole or orthotics can help the foot distribute pressure more evenly. Modifying the shoe with a stiff forefoot plate or a metatarsal bar can be done by a pedorthist. There are also special shoes available that have soles that can rock in such a way as to relieve pressure and pain on the joint. More serious cases may require surgery to remove the bony bumps or fuse the affected joint. In some cases, a joint replacement procedure may be need to restore toe and joint function and resolve the pain.

6

Blood Flow Conditions

To picture the network of blood vessels that make up the circulatory system of the legs and feet, visualize two upside down trees with trunks originating from the heart. One trunk is the aorta, the largest artery in the body. From this large trunk branch smaller and smaller vessels that reach throughout the body. This upside-down tree of branching arteries carries oxygen-filled blood away from the heart and throughout the body, including the legs and feet. The other trunk is the inferior vena cava, the largest vein in the body. The veins carry oxygen-depleted blood back to the heart. These two trees are connected at their farthest branches by capillaries—microscopic vessels so small that the individual blood cells have to flow through them single-file.

There is also another tree-like system in the body—the lymphatic system, which carries lymphatic fluid, or lymph, back to the heart. This is fluid that has seeped from the blood in the capillaries into the microscopic spaces between individual cells. Lymph funnels from these cells into lymph nodes and lymph vessels and is ultimately returned to the bloodstream. The lymphatic system is an important part of the body's immune system. Defects in this system can cause fluid to back up and the lower legs and ankles to swell.

Changes in blood flow can lead to a number of conditions of the lower legs and feet, such as varicose veins, pain, swelling, skin changes, hot or cold feet, slow healing, and open sores. Suspected blood flow disorders should be evaluated and treated by a physician because they can be an indication of serious conditions. Be aware of signs of blood flow changes and report them to you doctor

Some changes in blood flow occur inevitably with age. A decreased blood flow can result from accumulating plaques on blood vessel walls, calcification of vessels, or decreasing elasticity of the vessels themselves. In addition, the valves of the heart and veins that help maintain the flow of blood can falter.

The effects of aging on blood flow can be exacerbated by chronic disease and lifestyle factors. Hypertension, diabetes, and heart disease, all more common with age, are chronic diseases that contribute to blood flow changes in the feet and legs. Diet and nutrition, activity level of physical activity, and use of tobacco products are lifestyle issues that affect the health of the circulatory system.

Skin appearance and blood flow

Skin changes may be the most obvious evidence of decreased blood flow in the lower legs and feet. Changes in color, including paleness or blotchy patches of reddish, brownish, or bluish skin, are common indicators of diminished blood flow. In addition, brown spots can develop in areas that are prone to swelling, such as the lower legs or ankles. These spots, called hemosiderin deposits, occur when blood pools and deposits iron in the skin.

Changes in skin texture also occur when the skin is not adequately supplied with blood flow. The skin becomes thinner and drier, in severe cases taking on the appearance of rice paper. Or the skin may become inflamed or even break down, producing sores and ulcers. (This condition is known as stasis dermatitis and, as the name suggests, results from little or no blood flow to the dermis, or skin.) Other notable changes include decreased hair growth and a decreased ability to sweat.

As suggested above, the major consequence of decreased blood flow to the skin is that it thins, weakens, and becomes inflamed. This makes the skin more prone to injury, less able to heal, and more vulnerable to infection. In the worst cases of restricted blood flow, the skin can ulcerate or become gangrenous.

Toenails can also be affected by circulation disorders. With decreased blood flow, toenails can become thick, yellow, and brittle. In severe cases, they can loosen or even fall off. Toenail changes related to poor circulation can mimic or precede the appearance of fungal toenails, which is why circulation disorders must always be considered when fungal infections of the toenails are suspected.

Calf pain (deep vein thrombosis, or DVT)

A very serious circulatory condition of the lower legs is called deep vein thrombosis, or DVT. A DVT is a blood clot in a vein. It most commonly occurs in the calves. A DVT can cause pain, swelling, warmth, and redness in the affected area. Of greatest concern, though, is that the clot has the potential to break away from the blood vessel wall and travel to the lungs or heart, causing a life-threatening embolism. The risk factors for deep vein thrombosis are:

- recurrent or ongoing swelling
- physical trauma
- sitting or being immobile for long periods
- smoking
- high blood pressure
- high cholesterol

If your feet or legs swell when you travel, try wearing compression stockings on your trips.

While most calf pain is not caused by a DVT, it's best to be safe. See a doctor immediately if you suspect you may have a clot, especially if the symptoms described above persist or increase in severity. Never board a plane or embark on a long car ride if you are experiencing calf pain without first consulting a physician. There is always the potential for the DVT to dislodge and cause an embolism.

Compression stockings can be worn to minimize the risk of DVT. By maintaining an even compression of the lower legs, the risk of pooling and clotting is diminished. Physicians will prescribe compression stockings for those who may be at risk. Over-the-counter compression stockings are also available for use by people immobilized by an illness, injury, or other medical condition.

Edema (swelling)

Edema, also called swelling, occurs when fluid accumulates in a localized area of the body. Edema can be caused by inflammation and by circulatory changes. Some common causes of edema in the feet, ankles, or lower legs include:

- age-related changes in blood flow
- arthritis
- a blood clot (deep vein thrombosis, or DVT)
- dysfunctional venous valves
- gout
- heart disease
- infection
- injury or surgery
- lymphatic system disorders
- medication
- poor nutrition
- sitting or lying for long periods (such as when traveling or convalescing)
- standing for long periods
- varicose veins
- vascular disease

Moderate to severe swelling of the lower legs and feet can make it difficult to wear shoes or socks, or even to walk, and may indicate a serious illness. If left untreated, edema can cause the skin to deteriorate, making it thinner, less elastic, and more easily injured. In the worst cases, the skin will start to tear open and form weeping sores or ulcers that do not heal.

Treatment for edema

Any swelling that persists for more than a couple days should be seen by a medical professional. Swelling that is associated with pain should be seen right away. The first step for treating swelling is to have a podiatrist or medical doctor diagnose what's causing it. Then, that specific cause—illness, condition, or injury—can be addressed.

For minor cases, exercise, elevation, and the use of compression stockings are often all that is needed to alleviate or control the swelling. Compression stockings can be found in most pharmacies. Medical grade compression stockings offer a higher level of compression for moderate to severe swelling, but must be prescribed by a doctor and custom-fitted. In more severe cases, treatment may involve medications, changes in diet, the use of compression bandages, and physical therapy.

Walking pain (intermittent claudication, or IC)

The muscles of the lower legs require more oxygen when moving than resting. If the flow of blood to the legs is reduced, the muscles don't have enough oxygen to meet the increased demand of walking, and pain results. Because the calf muscles are relatively large, they demand a lot of oxygen and are often the first muscles to become painful when blood flow to the legs is reduced.

Walking pain caused by a reduction in blood flow to the muscles of the leg is called intermittent claudication, or IC. People suffering from IC usually describe episodes of pain after walking a certain distance—often one or two city blocks. The pain stops with rest, then resumes again with walking. The cause of the decreased blood flow is most often arterial disease. Those who suspect they have IC should see a physician for evaluation, diagnosis, and treatment.

Peripheral arterial disease (PAD)

Peripheral arterial disease, or PAD, refers to a group of disorders marked by decreased blood flow to the lower legs. This decreased blood flow can be caused by, among other things, diabetes, heart disease, hypertension, and smoking. PAD is more common in older populations; the risk for PAD increases each decade after the age of forty.[10]

PAD causes a number of changes to the structures of the lower legs. The skin can atrophy, leading to dryness and slowed healing. In severe cases, ulcers or open sores can develop. Bone density can decrease, and muscles and the plantar fat pad can shrink, leading to less cushioning under the feet. More severe forms of PAD will cause cramping in the lower leg or foot muscles, cold or blue toes and, in some cases, calf pain when walking. (See "walking pain" on p. 97.)

As with any suspected vascular condition, PAD must be evaluated and treated by a physician. Fortunately, exercise, smoking cessation, cholesterol-lowering drugs, and aspirin therapy have all been shown to be effective in managing the less severe forms of this condition.

Varicose veins and spider veins

Often a family trait, varicose veins are enlarged superficial veins that can be seen through the skin of the lower legs. They are the result of dysfunctional valves in the deep veins that cause increased blood flow in the superficial veins (those immediately under the skin). This increased flow enlarges the veins, causing them to bulge and become prominent. While varicose veins are usually painless, in some cases they may be painful. The biggest complaint about varicose veins is their appearance, which many find unattractive.

Varicose veins should be evaluated by a physician. They are commonly treated by exercising, elevating the legs, and wearing compression stockings. More severe cases may require surgical treatment by a vascular surgeon. Creams and lotions sold over the counter or through the Internet for "varicose vein relief" are ineffective and should be avoided.

Cold feet (vasospastic disorders)

Some people are born with feet that are easily chilled in cooler temperatures. While this characteristic may be a nuisance, it isn't serious. Those affected with this tendency can easily warm their feet by turning up the heat, turning down the air conditioning, or wearing warmer socks and footwear.

A more significant form of cold sensitivity is a group of disorders referred to collectively as vasospastic disorders. Conditions such as Raynaud's disease/phenomenon, pernio, and frostbite can all cause the muscles around the small vessels in the feet to spasm. The spasm constricts the vessels, preventing warm blood from reaching the toes.

If you suspect that you may have a vasospastic disorder, you should see a physician. Severe cases may require prescription medications to promote blood flow.

Hot feet (erythermalgia)

Erythermalgia is a condition characterized by changes in the color of the toes or balls of the feet, accompanied by sensations of burning, pain, and heat. The symptoms may be set off by being exposed to heat or by sitting for long periods. Fortunately, the symptoms can be often be alleviated simply by cooling and elevating the feet. Aspirin can help treat the pain. This condition should be evaluated by a podiatrist or primary care doctor since it has been associated with other systemic conditions, such lupus and thrombocytopenia.

7

Nerve Conditions

The small cells that make up the human nervous system are plentiful early in life but are lost faster than they are replaced as we age. Many of the changes we notice later in life—loss of memory, balance, and muscle strength—are associated with the decline of the nervous system and begin, imperceptibly, around age thirty. Researchers are learning that it is possible to slow this natural decline by performing tasks that are both mentally and physically challenging, such as doing crossword puzzles and exercising regularly. But, in the end, these activities cannot stave off all disorders of the nervous system.

While this book encourages self-treatment for the most routine foot problems, nerve disorders require a high level of medical expertise and should, therefore, be evaluated and treated by medical professionals. The most common nerve disorders are described in this chapter, but this description is no substitute for an exam by a primary care doctor, podiatrist, or neurologist.

Nerve disorders and gait changes

Any nerve disorder can cause changes in walking gait and balance. As we walk, the nerves in our feet are constantly sending messages to the

Common Causes of Leg and Foot Numbness and Weakness

adverse drug reactions/interactions	nerve tissue injury/trauma
alcohol abuse	Parkinson's disease
celiac disease	peripheral vascular disease
chemotherapy side effects	Raynaud's disease/phenomenon
deep vein thrombosis (DVT)	residual effects of frostbite
dementia/Alzheimer's disease	restless leg syndrome
diabetes	spinal stenosis
fibromyalgia	stroke
Guillaume-Barré syndrome	swelling
multiple mycelia	vitamin B12 deficiency

brain about the surface we're walking on—its regularity, firmness, texture. This feedback triggers the body to make countless subtle adjustments to every step in order to adapt to the terrain, absorb impact, and maintain balance.

The human nervous system is programmed to move the body in ways that cause the least amount of pain, cost the least amount of energy, and are the most stable. Nerve disorders can interfere with this programming. Consider, for example, if you were to have numbness in your feet. Because the numbness would make it difficult for you to feel the walking surface, you might compensate by walking more slowly and taking wider steps. Walking this way can waste energy and increase step impact, subjecting the joints, bones, and soft tissues of the feet to more force. If the numbness were also masking pain from an injury, you could exacerbate the damage without even knowing it.

Nerve disorders can manifest themselves as numbness in a small area of the foot, such as a toe or the side of the foot. They can also manifest themselves as numbness, pain, or burning that shoots up or down the foot or leg, or electrical sensations that travel from the foot to the thigh or buttocks. When numbness occurs over a broader area, such as all the toes or the lower leg, or involves both feet, then the condition may be what we call peripheral neuropathy.

Peripheral neuropathy (PN)

Peripheral neuropathy is a condition where the nerves of the feet cause burning, tingling, or numbness. This condition can be caused by vitamin B12 deficiency, diabetes, circulation disorders, frostbite, chemotherapy drugs, and alcohol abuse. In one third of cases, there is no identifiable cause. Some studies have shown that peripheral neuropathy is more common later in life, so it may be, to some degree, a consequence of aging.

PN usually affects both feet simultaneously and can start in the toes, then spreading slowly upward to the ankles and, in severe cases, to the knees and above. The decreased sensation in the feet related to peripheral neuropathy can interfere with balance, making some sufferers more vulnerable to falling. Recent research suggests that wearing special vibrating insoles may help to stimulate the nerve endings in the feet to give the wearer the neurological information they need to maintain balance.[11] These insoles are still in development, but they may be available soon.

Some of those affected by peripheral neuropathy experience symptoms only at night. They describe hot or crawly sensations on their feet and lower legs that cause discomfort and make it difficult to sleep. Doctor-prescribed medications are available that can quiet these sensations.

The biggest concern with PN is that because of the decreased sensation in the feet, scrapes, blisters, or other problems can go unnoticed and untreated, eventually becoming infected and ulcerous. For this reason, wearing new shoes can be a real problem for people with peripheral neuropathy. It is important for those with peripheral neuropathy to break in new shoes gradually and to inspect their feet immediately after taking off their new shoes.

Those with PN should be under the regular care of their podiatrist who can follow their condition and monitor possible complications. PN sufferers should see a podiatrist at the first sign of blistering, sores, or infection of the feet. Podiatrists can also help manage the condition by, among other things, fabricating custom insoles that minimize the risk of ulcers.

Spinal nerve root compression (radiculopathy)

Numbness or weakness that affects only one foot or a part of the foot or the outside of the calf may be caused by a spinal nerve root compression, or radiculopathy. Like the vascular system, large nerves originating in the spinal column divide into smaller and smaller branches as they spread into the extremities. The nerve root is the part of the nerve that exits the spinal column. It can be compressed by a bulging disc or injured vertebra from the spine. Numbness or burning pain on the outside of the foot or outside of the lower leg, for example, may be caused by a compressed nerve in the lower back. Occasionally, this type of numbness is preceded by low-back pain or pain that shoots down the buttocks or thigh. The sciatic nerve, the largest nerve in the body, is commonly affected by nerve root compression. This specific type of nerve root compression is often called sciatica.

Occasionally the pain from a nerve root compression is worsened by standing or sitting for long periods of time, or by extending the leg. Often, leaning slightly forward, such as is done when pushing a shopping cart, can relieve the pain.

Restless leg syndrome (RLS)

Restless leg syndrome is a condition that is usually painless but can be very disruptive. It causes uncomfortable sensations in the legs, usually at night, which can only be relieved by moving, walking, or changing position. Most people who suffer from RLS complain of sleep disturbance and discomfort.

According to the National Institute of Neurological Disorders and Stroke (a division of the National Institutes of Health), the cause of RLS is unknown but there are some contributing factors. Those with peripheral neuropathy, diabetes, Parkinson's disease, iron deficiency, anemia, and kidney disease may be susceptible to RLS. In addition, certain medications, alcohol, caffeine, and tobacco can aggravate the symptoms of RLS.

There is no cure for RLS, so therapy is directed at alleviating the symptoms. For treatment, seek the care of a medical professional. You may be asked to make certain lifestyle changes or take certain oral medications to control the symptoms. Vitamin or dietary supplements may provide relief for some RLS sufferers.

Burning forefoot or toe pain (neuroma)

Burning pain or numbness in the toes may be caused by a condition called Morton's neuroma. It is most common between the third and fourth toes. Morton's neuroma is the result of an enlarged and inflamed nerve in the forefoot. Symptoms are usually triggered by long periods of walking and standing. They may worsen during certain activities or while wearing certain shoes. Morton's neuroma seems to be more common in those with wide feet, and may be the result of tight shoes squeezing the feet together, causing mechanical irritation to the nerve.

Relief can sometimes be achieved by removing the shoe and rubbing the painful area. But more commonly, treatment consists of anti-inflammatory therapy, footwear changes, insole modifications (like metatarsal pads), and, occasionally, cortisone injections or surgery to decompress or remove the nerve.

Neuritis

Neuritis is an inflammation of a nerve. Pressure on or injury to a nerve can cause it to become inflamed. For example, burning or numbness in the side of the big toe may be the result of the side of the shoe pressing against a bunion, which irritates the underlying nerve. Nerves can become trapped in scar tissue that has formed after an injury or near a surgical incision. Also, pain on the top of the foot can be caused by nerves aggravated by tying the shoes too tight.

Patients with neuritis often describe "shooting" or "electric" pain, "pins and needles," or feeling "jabbed with a hot poker." In severe cases, even the weight of a sheet or pressure from stockings can cause extreme pain.

Neuritis can sometimes be difficult to differentiate from other nerve disorders. People experiencing its symptoms should visit a doctor for evaluation and treatment. Identifying and addressing sources of pressure, such as shoes, scars, or previous injuries, is important to treating neuritis. Icing, massage, and anti-inflammatory treatment can help relieve some of the discomfort.

Tarsal tunnel syndrome

Carpal tunnel syndrome is a condition that most people have heard of. It results from the compression of the nerve that passes over the carpal bones and enters the opening, or carpal tunnel, at the front of the wrist. The tarsal tunnel is a similar structure in the foot. When the nerve is compressed, it causes burning or sharp pain in the inside ankle or arch area of the foot. Occasionally, it will cause pain or numbness that extends all the way to the big toe. Tarsal tunnel syndrome can be caused by an injury, such as an ankle sprain, or it can occur gradually as the result of a weak arch that collapses too much, increasing pressure on the nerve inside the tunnel.

Treatment consists of supporting the foot and arch to decrease pressure in the tunnel and to lower repetitive tension on the nerve. Occasionally, cortisone injections may be used to relieve inflammation and aid other treatment measures. As with carpal tunnel syndrome, more serious cases of tarsal tunnel syndrome may require corrective surgery.

Weakness and drop foot

Weakness of the feet or legs may be hard to detect at first. In fact, sometimes the first sign of weakness may be occasional tripping or an altered walking style. Over time, however, weakness becomes more pronounced and obvious. Drop foot, for example, is a condition where the muscles on the front of the lower leg are greatly weakened. Sufferers of drop foot lose the ability to pull the toes up while the leg is moving forward during walking. The toes then drop, which causes the affected individual to have to lift the knee higher in order to get the toes to clear the ground.

Weakness of the feet or legs may be temporary or permanent and can be caused by stroke, spinal cord injury, leg fracture, spinal nerve root compression, spinal stenosis, a nerve tumor, nerve trauma, peroneal nerve palsy, or as a complication of knee surgery. In addition to weakness and altered gait, there may be numbness and pain.

Doctors typically treat drop foot with a rigid, plastic, lower-leg shell called an ankle foot orthosis. It can help those with drop foot walk by preventing the toes from pointing down as the foot swings forward. Physical therapy may be ordered once the cause of the weakness is identified, so that a gait retraining and strengthening program can be started. A word of caution: Weakness can be caused by a number of medical conditions, some of them serious, so any type of weakness, including drop foot, should be evaluated by a physician.

8

Shoes

To a foot in a shoe, the whole world seems paved with leather
—*The Hitopadesa,* 500 A.D.

Accccording to the American Podiatric Medical Association, 85 percent of the U.S. population will seek medical care for foot pain at some point in their lives. In cultures that do not wear shoes, however, such as those in parts of Africa and India, less than 10 percent of the population will seek medical care for foot pain.[12] Granted, health care access is more limited in these countries, but it has been well documented that shoe-wearing populations are more prone to chronic foot problems. The disparity in foot problems between barefoot and shod cultures shows that wearing shoes tends to make feet weaker and more susceptible to injury than going barefoot. One researcher, after observing barefoot persons in China and India, went so far as to conclude that shoes were "the cause of most of the ailments of the human foot."[13]

Walking barefoot allows the feet to function naturally, forcing the muscles to expand and contract, and the joints to bend and stretch to absorb step impact. This, in turn, promotes muscle strength and healthy joint alignment. Conversely, wearing shoes can inhibit the natural function of the feet by providing artificial cushioning and support, constricting the feet into unnatural positions and limiting air flow around the skin and nails. Because of this, muscles weaken, the range of motion in the joints is restricted, alignment of the toes can start to change, and skin and nail conditions can develop. The feet grow dependent on footwear, are deformed by footwear, and become less resistant to injury and disease.

Does this mean that we should all be walking barefoot? Perhaps, in an ideal world, but for most of us this is not a possibility. For one thing, we are continually forced to walk on artificially hard surfaces, such as asphalt, concrete, and tile, from which our feet require some sort of cushioning and support. For another, our culture demands that we wear shoes in public places for reasons of social decorum and public health. Most importantly, we need shoes to protect our feet from injury. Indeed, originally shoes were tools that protected the feet from weather, climate, terrain, and other hazards. But over time, many kinds of shoes have become primarily fashion accessories and have lost their protective functions, weakening and even deforming the feet they were once intended to protect.

What, then, can we do in today's shoe-dependent cultures to promote healthy feet? The most important thing we can do is to wear shoes that fit well and provide the proper amount of cushioning and support. A study of foot measurements in subjects 65 and older found that two-thirds were wearing shoes that were too narrow.[14] Other research has shown that overcushioned shoes do not protect from step impact and, in some cases, can even increase impact when compared to firmer footwear.[15] Many foot problems can be aggravated or even caused by shoes. Often, a significant amount of foot pain can be alleviated simply by switching to proper footwear.

Finding appropriate footwear, however, can be a daunting task. Many people are confused by the conflicting advice they receive about shoes. I have had patients come to their first appointment carrying bags of shoes. They can list for each pair who recommended the shoes and why. A friend suggested this pair because it worked for her. A doctor suggested another pair because the brand comes in five widths. The catalog guaranteed relief with yet another pair. A well-meaning shoe store employee recommended still another. And so on.

To compound matters, the sheer number of shoe models available can leave a person overwhelmed and puzzled where to begin. Purchasing shoes forty years ago was a simpler task. There were basically three categories of shoes: work shoes, dress shoes, and sport shoes. Most sport shoes, or sneakers, had rubber soles and canvas uppers, and were intended for use in any sport. There were no specialized shoes for running, walking, aerobics, or cross training. (The term "cross training" wasn't even around forty years ago.) Today, shoppers confront countless models of shoes for nearly every conceivable purpose. Manufacturers have introduced cushioning innovations such as air units, gel pads, and light foam. Yet despite these "advances" in footwear design, foot pain and injuries are as common today as they were in the 1960s.

A recent Internet search for "walking shoes" resulted in hits for 602 different models!

So what are proper shoes? In the simplest terms, proper shoes are those that allow the foot to function as naturally as possible. They also offer a combination of good stability and appropriate cushioning. Proper shoes do not force the foot into unnatural positions or shapes. These basic guidelines apply to all shoe wearers, but especially to older adults and those experiencing foot problems.

Unfortunately, it isn't always immediately clear what is meant by normal foot function, good stability, and appropriate cushioning. This chapter, then, will attempt to clarify these guidelines and other matters related to footwear, while providing information to help you choose the best shoes for your particular needs.

The myth of cushioning

Many people assume that foot problems can be addressed by wearing softer, more cushioned shoes. This is not the case. In fact, too much cushioning can actually cause more problems than it solves. And if cushioning isn't combined with stabilizing features, the feet can be strained by the very cushioning that is supposedly providing relief. Here's why. Cushioning is inversely related to stability. The human body is amazingly efficient at absorbing step impact if there is good stability underfoot. When you step on excessive cushioning, however, your foot's ability to absorb impact is compromised, and there is no stable foundation to push back against. Simply, then, more cushioning means less stability.

Let's explore this relationship further. Though seemingly counterintuitive, too much cushioning increases the strain on the foot and compromises stability. Think of walking on sand. Few would argue that sand is softer that concrete. Walking for long periods on sand, however, takes a lot of effort. Sand is an unstable walking surface. It collapses as the foot pushes against it, and this results in the feet, ankles, and knee joints all experiencing higher workloads. While overly cushioned shoes aren't nearly as unstable as sand, the effect is similar.

Excessively cushioned shoes can also defeat the nerves of the feet because they make it more difficult to sense the walking surface. Much the way that gloves interfere with the sense of touch in the hands, cushioning in shoes interferes with the sense of touch in the soles. There are thousands of nerves in the soles of the feet that provide feedback to the brain to assist in walking, running, and maintaining balance. If the nerves are disturbed by artificially unstable surfaces (i.e., excessive cushioning), they send inaccurate information to the brain.

This isn't to say that shoes shouldn't have cushioning. Cushioning moderate enough to prevent the foot from collapsing the shoe to one side or the other, combined with such stabilizing features as arch supports, medial posts, and a straighter shape to the shoe's outsole are qualities of a good shoe with proper fit.

What is the best shoe?

I am constantly being asked by my patients, "What is the best shoe?" I wish there were a simple answer, but there a just too many variables in individual needs to be addressed in one magical shoe. Arch height, foot shape, previous injuries or surgeries, and comfort are but a few of the factors that influence which shoe will work best for you. The "best shoe" is the shoe that fits the foot well and supports it properly for the use it is being put to.

Curiously, I have never been asked, "What is the worst shoe?" My guess is that this is because the answer is fairly obvious. Many types of dress shoes, including high heels and cowboy boots, are bad for your feet. Certain foot problems can be directly attributed to the long-term use of high-heeled, narrow-toed shoes, including hammertoes, bunions, corns, and ingrown toenails. Having said this, I realize that in our culture we are expected at times to wear these types of shoes. My recommendation is to spend as much of your time as possible wearing shoes that fit well and feel good.

What are the qualities of shoes that make them fit well and feel good? Not every shoe that offers good support and cushioning is comfortable for everyone. Ask one hundred people to define comfort as it relates to shoes, and you'll get one hundred different answers. Some say comfort is the result of a good fit. Others feel that comfort is due to support. Still others feel that comfort comes from a shoe that feels "natural" when they walk. Shoe companies have commissioned scientific studies hoping to unlock the secrets of comfort, but have found no conclusive results.[16] Comfort is ultimately subjective. Doctors, shoe clerks, manufacturers, and others can suggest what makes for comfortable shoes, but, in the end, the only authority on comfort is you.

Special considerations for women's shoes

By some counts, 80 percent of visits to podiatrists are made by women. Anatomically, there is very little difference between men's and women's feet. However, there are significant differences between the shoes that men and women wear. Men generally are less tolerant of shoes that are uncomfortable, while many women are willing to sacrifice comfort in favor of style. Also, women often have more difficulty finding wide or large sizes. Many women know that painful

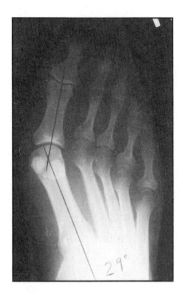 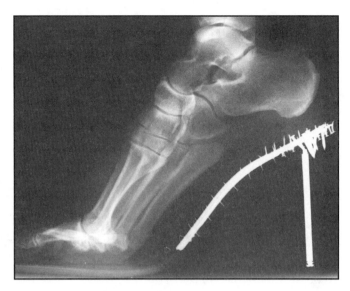

Above: X-rays of a 35-year-old patient wearing a 3-1/2-inch heel. Note in the X-ray on the left how her toes are pinched together and she appears to have a bunion at the crossing lines by her big toe joint. The shadow of the shoe's pointed toe is seen at the top of the X-ray.

Below: The same patient standing barefoot.

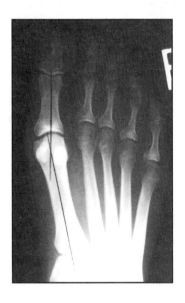 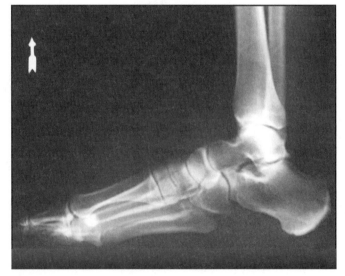

feet are the price one pays for wearing many kinds of fashionable shoes. Indeed, a survey of women on shoe-related pain conducted by Carol Frey, M.D., and colleagues in 1993[17] found that

- 80 percent of women reported significant foot pain while wearing shoes.
- 88 percent wore shoes that were too small as measured by an orthopedic surgeon.
- 76 percent had foot deformities, with bunions and hammertoes being most common.
- 59 percent wore uncomfortable shoes on a daily basis.
- 79 percent had not had their feet measured in the last five years when buying shoes.
- most women first experienced foot-related problems in their twenties.

For centuries, cultural influences around the world have forced or encouraged women to accentuate their legs and disguise their feet. In

A Shoe Clerk's Perspective

I worked in shoe stores while a podiatry student and have seen first hand how difficult it can be to convince some women that they are wearing shoes that are too small for their feet. In my experience, many women have become so accustomed to tight, constricting shoes, that when they wear properly fitting shoes, they are convinced that the shoes feel "sloppy." Both as a student and as a practicing podiatrist, numerous women have insisted to me that their shoe width was double-A or triple-A when they clearly needed footwear two or three sizes wider. As a shoe clerk, I had to give them what they wanted, and they almost always wanted the shoes that were too small. As a podiatrist, I can now advise both women and men that their foot pain will only get worse if they insist on wearing poorly fitting shoes.

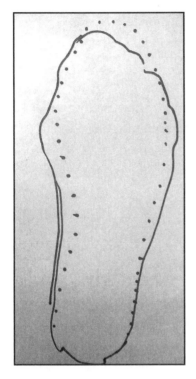

In order to illustrate how poorly her shoes fit, I made a tracing of the patient's foot below. The solid line represents her foot while standing and the dotted line represents the shape of the shoe she was wearing. Her foot was three-quarters of an inch wider than her shoe.

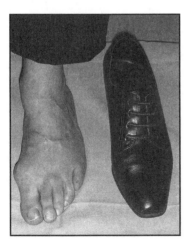

China, for example, foot binding was common for hundreds of years until finally outlawed in 1911. Girls as young as three had their feet bound with strips of cloth to restrict growth so that their dainty feet would resemble a lotus flower. The results, however, were pointed, three-inch-long feet and a lifetime of agonizing foot pain and disability.

While today's fashionable shoes—often pointed and high heeled—do not cause the profound deformities of foot binding, many do constrict the feet and contribute to painful conditions such as bunions, hammertoes, corns, ingrown toenails, and pinched nerves.[18] The narrow platform and elevated heel also puts more strain on the ball of the feet and interferes with balance when compared to flat shoes.[19]

Pointed toes and high heels are only part of the problem for women's feet. Almost 90 percent of women wear shoes that are too small. Again, Dr. Frey found that the average woman wears shoes that are one-half inch to one inch too narrow and a half size to a full size too short. Many woman could achieve a tremendous amount of relief from most painful foot conditions simply by wearing shoes with more room. In fact, the most important step in treating most foot conditions is to ensure that shoes fit properly.

Many older men also wear shoes that are too small for their feet, but this may be more due to a lack of availability of shoes that fit their changing feet than to improper size selection.[20] It may sound obvious, but the best way to distinguish between shoes that are "good" and shoes that are "bad" is that good shoes do not cause foot pain. Generally, fashion or dress shoes are the most likely to cause foot pain. For this reason, every woman should have at least one pair of comfortable walking or casual shoes.

Increasing demand for "comfort footwear" (a recently coined term referring to footwear that emphasizes comfort over fashion) reflects shifting emphasis in the U.S. for shoes that provide relief from foot pain. Recently, there has been a marked increase in sales of sandals and athletic shoes to women. Women are becoming more involved in fitness activities and are buying shoes that help them stay active. Wider social acceptance of healthier shoes for women would contribute to dramatic improvement of women's foot health.

Can women's shoes be stylish, fit well, and be good for the feet? Unfortunately, it is extremely difficult to combine style and comfort. Some manufacturers of footwear are attempting to make shoes for women that are both healthy and fashionable. Dr. Taryn Rose is an orthopedic surgeon who has developed a line of footwear that provides comfort without sacrificing style, and Munro American produces high-heeled and dress shoes with such comfort features as width sizing and removable foot beds. Keep in mind that high heels and narrow, pointed shoes will never be good for the feet. Period. However, high heels that are sized properly are "less bad" for the feet than poorly fitting high heels. The bottom line is that shoes should not cause pain.

Both men and women can make more informed choices when buying shoes after they've gained an understanding of the structure of shoes and how certain shoe characteristics may affect their feet. Such basic things as shoe shape and construction materials can have profound effects on the health of the feet.

Shoe construction

As previously noted, there are thousands of shoe types and styles available on the shelves of America's shoe stores. New Balance, one of the largest manufacturers of athletic shoes, for example, makes more than twenty different models of walking shoes.[21] It's easy to become overwhelmed when facing all these choices.

Fortunately, it is not necessary to evaluate thousands of shoes. It's much simpler to learn some of the basics of shoe construction. By learning about the basics of shoe construction and knowing your personal preferences and unique needs, you can focus on identifying the shoes that are best for you. The basics of shoe construction include:

- upper
- toe box
- outsole
- midsole
- heel cup
- insole
- shoe last

Upper

The shoe's upper is the most important part of the shoe. Think of it as the part of the shoe that "receives" the foot. The upper is what secures the shoe to the foot and is the most visible part of the shoe. Combined with the outsole, the upper creates the shape of the shoe and provides varying amounts of volume to accommodate the foot. The upper is important because it affects so many aspects of shoe quality—fit, protection, durability, and breathability. In a "good" shoe, the upper wraps the foot gently, holds it securely, protects it from the environment, and allows enough air movement that the skin can "breathe." In a "bad" shoe, the upper squeezes the foot into an unnatural shape, increases the risk of falling by being either too tight or loose, provides inadequate protection from the environment, and restricts air movement, contributing to skin and nail problems.

Upper construction and materials

An upper may be made of leather, synthetic leather, canvas, mesh fabric, elastic fabric, plastic, rubber, or foam. The function of the shoe, of course, influences which materials are selected for the upper. Athletic shoes are usually made from more breathable materials, such as vented leather or mesh. Shoes for wet or cold weather activities will have rubber, treated leather, or waterproof fabric uppers. Quality upper materials provide some ability to stretch or give without losing their durability. Stiff leather or hard plastics in the upper of the shoe can cause blisters and foot pain. Recently, uppers made from durable but elastic fabrics have become available. These types of uppers are great for those with wide feet, bunions, or hammertoes. While not as durable as leather, the fabric can secure the shoe to the foot while minimizing pressure on the top of the foot.

Too often we overlook the seams of the upper when we are evaluating shoes. Uppers can be comprised of a number of panels of fabric sewn together. The seams that join these panels can cause irritation if they lie over a bony prominence, such as a bunion or hammertoe. Some seams affect how the shoe flexes as the heel is lifted. The seams are also a common area of failure in shoes that are excessively worn. When trying on new shoes, be aware of where the seams lie and avoid shoes with seams in sensitive areas. For example, if you have a bunion, this would be directly over your big toe joint.

Upper volume

Sometimes we get so caught up in thinking of shoes in terms of length and width that we overlook the fact that shoes also have volume. If we were to fill both a size 10 walking shoe and a size 10 dress shoe with water and compare the volumes, we would find that the walking shoe holds more water. Even within the same category we might find significant differences in volume between different models and manufacturers. A walking shoe with a larger-volume upper will fit and feel significantly different than a walking shoe with less volume. The volume of the upper is influenced by the toe box shape, shoe last, upper depth, lacing system, and elastic properties of the upper material. Those with wide feet, bunions, arthritis, diabetes, and swelling often are more comfortable in shoes that have a more voluminous upper.

Lacing and closure type

Most shoes are secured to the foot with some sort of closure system. Laces, of course, are the most common, but zippers, buckles, snaps, elastic bands, and hook-and-loop closures such as Velcro are also used. Zippers and snaps tend to be the least versatile and most restrictive types of closure, while laces and hook-and-loop straps tend to be the most versatile and least restrictive. Shoes that slip on without any form of closure system cannot secure the foot inside the shoe or adjust the fit of the shoe.

The shape of the opening for the laces or other closure type is as important as the closure type itself. Generally, longer openings provide more versatility and a more secure fit. Skilled shoe repair shops or pedorthists can modify a shoe's closure type. Some common foot problems can be relieved by using certain lacing patterns.

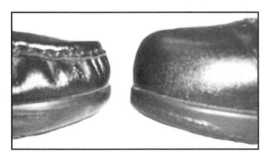

A toe box of conventional depth on the left compared to a toe box with additional depth on the right.

Toe box

The toe box can vary in shape from extremely narrow and pointed to very round and wide. A pointed toe box is unnatural and forces the toes together, while rounder toe boxes tend to follow the natural shape of the foot. While not as common as pointed and rounded toe boxes, square toe boxes are also usually better for the toes than pointed shapes.

Though often overlooked, the depth of the toe box can, for some people, be the most important part of a good fit. Those with painful

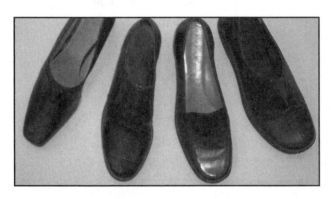

Above are some examples of toe box shapes, progressing from a squared-off point on the left to a rounded roomy toe box on the right. The volume of each shoe increases from left to right.

corns, hammertoes, or swollen feet should wear shoes with extra depth. Depth is not a part of shoe measurement the way that length and width are. Brands such as San Antonio Shoes (SAS) and Drew provide a measurement of toe depth along with length and width. Your podiatrist may recommend this type of shoe, or a well-trained shoe salesperson will be familiar with which shoe models are designed for additional depth.

Outsole

The outsole is the bottom of the shoe and is usually made from rubber, synthetics, or leather. The most supportive shoes will have rubber or vinyl outsoles, which provide cushioning, flexibility, and traction on many surfaces.

Midsole

The midsole is sandwiched between the outsole and the upper. This layer provides most of the cushioning and support of the feet. Not all shoes have midsoles. Shoes without midsoles do not have much, if any, support and offer only minimal cushioning. Most dress shoes, for example, do not have a midsole, while almost all athletic shoes do.

Heel cup

The heel cup is, as its name suggests, designed to hold the heel in place. It should secure the heel snugly but not so snugly as to cause blisters. Heel cups vary in depth. A deep heel cup secures the heel better than a shallow one. Many dress shoes have shallow heel cups, while athletic shoes tend to have deep heel cups.

Insoles

Insoles line the foot bed. They may be made of leather, foam, fabric, or cork and are usually glued or sewn into the shoe. One of the best footwear innovations of the last few years is the removable insole.

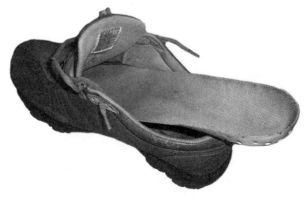

Many makes of comfort shoes have removable insoles.

Removable insoles are not attached to the shoe. They were initially found only in athletic shoes but have become more common in casual shoes and even some dress shoes. The ability to remove the insole makes it easier to customize shoes by adding supportive devices, such as metatarsal pads or arch pads, or by replacing the insoles with custom orthotics or more supportive insoles. The best shoe insoles add cushioning and arch support. Insoles can easily be changed, used in multiple pairs of shoes, and modified to treat certain foot problems. Some models of dress shoes, such as those made by Rockport, Ecco, and others, offer removable insoles. Better-quality casual shoes and athletic shoes will have removable insoles. If you have foot pain and are very active, I strongly recommend that you wear shoes with removable insoles.

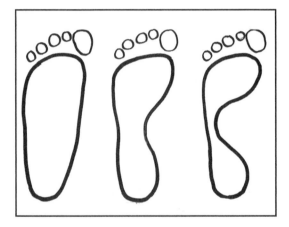

A flat foot, neutral foot, and high-arched foot (above, left to right) match up with a straight last, semi-straight last, and curved last, respectively (below, left to right).

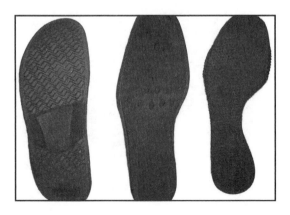

Shoe last

The last refers to the shape of a shoe's outsole. There are three basic types: curved, semicurved, and straight. For the best support, it is important to match the shoe last to the foot shape. The more curved the last, the less support there is under the arch of the foot. A flat or low arch matches up best with a straight last, while a medium to moderately low arch matches up best with a semistraight last. A high arch is best paired with a curved last. In my experience, too many people wear curved last shoes that cause their feet to collapse excessively and strain the foot and ankle.

Characteristics of quality shoes

Well-made shoes will have some features in common:

- leather or breathable mesh uppers
- soft lining with no hard or poorly located seams
- removable insoles
- slip-resistant outsole
- flexibility at the forefoot

Poor-quality upper materials do not breathe as well as soft leather or mesh uppers, are not as durable, and can deform or break apart sooner. A soft lining, without irritating or poorly placed seams, will decrease the risk of blistering, provide more comfort, and help pull moisture away from the skin. Removable insoles are excellent for making modifications to the shoe and can be replaced by more supportive insoles if necessary. Slip-resistant outsoles minimize the risk of falls on wet or slippery surfaces.

Shoes need to bend where the feet bend, and they need to be stiff where the feet do not bend. For example, shoes should be flexible under the ball of the feet so that the toes can bend naturally as the heel lifts. Instead of flexing under the ball of the feet, poorly made shoes may flex under the arch, straining the foot muscles and plantar fascia. A good test to see where a shoe flexes is to grasp the shoe with both hands—one at the toe and one at the heel—and force it to bend. A shoe that does not flex at the toes will strain your foot. Some shoes are so flimsy that they can practically be folded with only one hand. If you have an arthritic condition of the forefoot, stiffer shoes may protect your feet better than more flexible shoes.

Recommended shoe styles

Although all shoes are similar in terms of construction and materials, there a certain styles of shoes that are better for our feet than others. The shoe styles listed below offer features that promote healthy feet. Keep in mind that these categories are broad, and some shoes cross between categories.

Casual shoes

Casual shoes are a broad category of shoes suitable for everyday use. For many people they represent a compromise, being more formal than athletic shoes, yet less formal and more comfortable than dress shoes. They tend to have less restrictive construction than dress shoes but more support. Typically, casual shoes accommodate insoles better than dress shoes. The best casual shoes have removable insoles, leather uppers, and durable rubber outsoles.

Additional-depth shoes

Additional-depth shoes are casual shoes that have more room from top to bottom. The extra depth can decrease pressure on toes and allow for custom orthotics or insoles. Better-quality shoes in this category have a seamless, padded construction with soft leather or flexible fabric uppers. Footwear manufacturers who specialize in additional-depth shoes include Aetrex, SAS, Drew, and P.W. Minor. These shoes are especially recommended for those with diabetes, neuropathy, hammertoes, or swelling and are typically found in stores that specialize in comfort shoes.

Athletic shoes

In addition to fitness activities, athletic shoes are beneficial for everyday use by active people. Running and walking shoes are suitable for all around use, but active individuals who participate in a sport more than once a week should wear sport-specific shoes when playing. Those who play tennis regularly, for example, should be wear court shoes. I do not recommend canvas sneakers if you have any sort of foot pain. They are heavier than most other athletic shoes yet offer less support and cushioning. If you have an ankle injury, high-top shoes and boots offer additional ankle support.

Sandals and clogs

Many people prefer the open feeling of sandals and clogs to the more restricted feeling of lace-up shoes. Like lace-up shoes, however, there are some sandals and clogs that are more supportive than others. "Flip flops," or thong-type sandals, offer little or no support and can easily catch on stairs or uneven surfaces, causing the wearer to trip. More supportive sandals can be a good alternative to house slippers for casual wear at home. An increasing number of shoe manufacturers are making sandals that can accommodate insoles and custom orthotics. Still, if you have decreased sensation in your feet or problems with balance, you should wear any type of sandal with caution, as debris can get under the foot more easily and the less secure upper can contribute to slips and falls.

Clogs are better in cooler climates and offer more protection than sandals. Also, clogs are generally better able to accommodate insoles or orthotics than sandals. The shoe company Crocs makes a foam clog that provides cushioning and plenty of toe room and is comfortable for both indoor and outdoor use.

Why I Don't Recommend Only One Brand of Shoes

While there are a number of shoe manufacturers who have well-deserved reputations for making quality products, I never focus on one particular brand when recommending shoes. Nike is arguably the most recognized brand in the world, but despite their reputation for quality products and endorsements by famous athletes, buying Nike shoes does not guarantee that you will get a better fit or support for your feet. Instead of seeking out one brand, look at different models by different manufacturers. Each manufacturer will make some shoes that work well for you and some that don't. It's worth taking some time to find those that do work well for you.

While slip-on footwear offers ease and convenience, patients who have problems with balance or a history of falls should avoid footwear that does not have some way to secure the heel. The loose or open heel of some sandals and clogs can increase the risk of falling or slipping.

Slippers or house shoes

Footwear worn inside the house can be a crucial but often overlooked piece of the cause and treatment puzzle of foot pain. Most slippers are designed primarily to keep the feet warm and provide very little cushioning. They are not very supportive and often not very durable. In fact, some foot pain can be directly attributed their lack of support and protection. Since slippers are made to be slipped on, they tend to fit poorly and have been implicated in increased risk of falling. For those with foot pain, slippers or going barefoot around the house should be avoided, and more supportive footwear should be used instead.

New styles of footwear are becoming available for use around the house that represent a good alternative to slippers. Brands such as Haflinger and Crocs offer clog-style footwear that provides cushioning, support, and durability. Haflinger's clog has a supportive cork footbed and boiled wool upper, while Crocs have a unique one-piece construction of EVA, which is the same foam that cushions running shoes. This type of footwear will cost more than inexpensive slippers—between $30 and $100—but they are better for the feet than slippers and will outlast most slippers by years, making them a more healthy and economical choice.

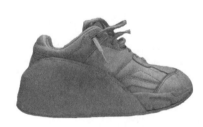

Above: This shoe has been modified with a medial buttress.

Below: The shoe on the right has been similarly modified to support a collapsing ankle.

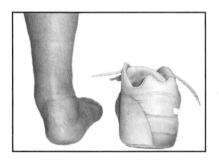

Modified shoes

Certified pedorthists can often make modifications to off-the-shelf shoes to accommodate and treat certain conditions. For example, a medial buttress is an addition to the arch side of the shoe. When skillfully applied, a medial buttress greatly improves the ability of the shoe to prevent a flat foot from collapsing off the edge of the shoe.

A certified pedorthist or shoe repair shop can also convert a lace-up shoe to a hook-and-loop closure system for those who may have difficulty tying laces. The change is relatively simple and inexpensive. Other types of modifications include adding a rocker bottom or metatarsal bars to relieve forefoot pain, adding lifts to balance out differences in leg length, and applying denser, more durable materials to areas of excessive wear.

Shoes that defy classification

Footwear innovations are continuously introduced. Unfortunately, most offer dubious benefits. Some innovations, such the MBT(Masai Barefoot Technology) shoes by Swiss Masai, however, can be helpful for those with arthritic feet and knees. Researchers have shown that these unique shoes help to strengthen muscles and improve ankle stability.[22] The shoes are a new twist on an old idea: rocker bottom shoes. Rocker bottom shoes have been used for decades to decrease strain on certain joints of the feet. The

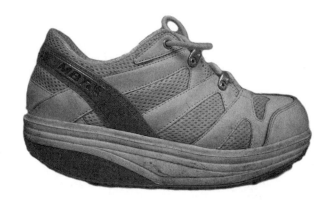

A Masai Barefoot Technology (MBT) shoe by Swiss Masai. Note the unique midsole shape.

MBT shoes have a rocker feature at the heel and at the toe. While these shoes have therapeutic benefits for some, they should not be worn by those who have poor balance.

Shoes with springs, such as those made by Z-Coil, have gained a following almost as much for their appearance as for their shock-absorbing ability. The large coiled spring in the heel can absorb some step impact, but it also makes the shoe heavier than conventional footwear. Those who work in jobs that require long periods of standing seem to benefit from this type of footwear. Both Z-Coils and MBTs are more expensive than conventional footwear, and there is no guarantee that they will relieve foot or leg pain. But for some they may be worth the extra expense.

Earth shoes, which became popular in the 1970s, are another unique type of footwear. The distinguishing feature of earth shoes is the "negative" heel. The heel on an earth shoe is lower than the forefoot, which simulates how the heel might sink into a naturally soft surface such as sand or grass when walking. Earth shoes also feature straight lasts and round toe boxes that allow the feet to function in a more natural manner. Research on negative-heel shoes has shown that joint range of motion in hips, knees, and ankles is altered and foot pressures change as well. Some people can benefit from these changes.

Future Footwear

The future of footwear is quite promising. Shoes may soon have footbeds that mold to the contour of the sole and are treated to prevent the growth of bacteria and fungus. They may even contain computer sensors that adjust the cushioning of the shoes with every step. In fact, the technology for these features already exists and is in limited use. Adidas, for example, is using computer technology in one of its running shoes.

A process called "mass customization" is beginning to make custom footwear more affordable. A company called Otabo has introduced into retail settings a manufacturing process that scans the feet with a 3D laser and creates a mold, or last. Customers can then select the style, material and color of the custom shoes they want. The shoes are manufactured to specification, arriving by mail a few weeks after the order is placed. The mold is kept in storage so that future shoes can be ordered over the Internet as needed.

Shoes I don't recommend

I have not included dress shoes in the recommended styles. There are three main reasons why I do not recommend them:

1. Women's dress shoes (more so than men's) force the feet into unnatural positions and only make most foot problems worse.
2. Because of their restrictive shape, dress shoes cannot accommodate a supportive insole, which is often necessary to treat painful foot conditions.
3. Most dress shoes cannot be stretched or modified enough to improve their function.

Granted, some dress shoes are better for the feet than others, and more manufacturers are making dress shoes that offer comfort as well as style. But overall, casual and athletic shoes provide a much healthier alternative.

I would also advise you to be skeptical of shoe manufacturers who claim that their products are "guaranteed to relieve foot pain" or offer "revolutionary technology" or "built-in orthotics." Certain shoes, in certain cases, can provide pain relief, improve alignment, or prevent fatigue, but there is no shoe that can provide all those things for all people. You may hear some manufacturers go so far as to claim that their shoes will resolve migraine headaches and sciatica. While it's possible for hip, back, and neck pain to be relieved to some degree by wearing certain types of footwear, I always give my patients this rule of thumb: the farther your pain is from your feet anatomically, the less likely the type of shoes you wear will help relieve the pain.

Where to buy shoes

It's not always easy to find a shoe store with a well-trained staff, a broad selection, and a reasonable return policy. Those who live in rural areas or small towns will have to be especially resourceful in finding places to shop for shoes. Asking friends, neighbors, medical professionals, or family members where they shop for shoes may be the best starting point.

Shoe retailers

As with any commercial product, it is always best to buy shoes from an experienced and reputable seller. Most communities have reputable shoe stores with staff who are willing to spend the time necessary to help you find good shoes. Many independent shoe retailers and regional chains have found a niche by leaving fashion shoes to the large department stores and boutique shops and focusing on comfort and athletic shoes. In my experience, these retailers generally provide good customer service.

Wherever you shop, be cautious and use your best judgment when buying shoes and shoe products. Some retailers encourage their sales associates to upsell; some make diagnoses they are unqualified to make. Walk away from stores that attempt to sell you products you don't need, and walk quickly away from those whose employees attempt to diagnose a foot problem. The only people qualified to make a diagnosis or offer treatment options are medical professionals.

Some shoe stores have a certified pedorthist on staff. In much the same way that a pharmacist fills prescriptions and offers advice about medications, a certified pedorthist can evaluate customers' feet and make recommendations for shoes, insoles, and shoe modifications. Many podiatrists and orthopedists rely on certified pedorthists to help their patients with their foot problems.

Discount "big box" stores and discount chains

There's no getting around it: quality shoes are expensive, and I would be remiss to ignore the fact that some budgets do not allow for the purchase of higher-priced shoes. Lower-priced footwear can be found at discount "big box" stores such as Target and Wal-Mart and national discount chains such as Payless Shoes and Famous Footwear. These stores offer shoes at heavily discounted prices, and while the quality may be variable, you can find shoes with the features you need if you know what you're looking for. A good starting point would be to bring along your most comfortable shoes and look for shoes that have a similar shape, support, and cushioning. Don't make your buying decisions based solely on price; often shoes that cost a bit more are a better value in the long run.

Footcare centers

Footcare centers are a new type of retail shoe store that, as their name suggests, sell more types of products than the traditional shoe store. In addition to shoes, most offer a wide range of footcare products. Footcare centers may be part of a national chain, like Foot Solutions, or a local retailer, like the New York-based Eneslow Foot Comfort Center. Some footcare centers use computers to scan your feet for more precise sizing, fitting, and customizing. (Keep in mind, however, that computers or high-tech gadgets are no substitute for a knowledgeable sales staff.) The best footcare centers will have a pedorthist on staff.

Some footcare centers specialize more in insoles and arch supports than shoes. The prices charged for these insoles can vary widely from retailer to retailer. Terms such as "custom fit" and "custom molded" may be used to describe insoles costing $90 to $300 or more. These premium-priced insoles may or may not be as helpful as a $30 to $50 off-the-shelf insole. In fact, I would not recommend spending more than $50 on any insole or orthotic, even if it's custom made, unless you have been diagnosed and specifically instructed to do so by a medical professional. Insoles are usually more difficult to return or exchange if they do not work. This is especially the case for custom devices. (Insoles and orthotics are discussed in more detail in the next chapter.)

Mail order and the Internet

Unless you are buying the exact brand, model, and size of a shoe you are familiar with (or are ordering a custom shoe from a laser foot scan), you should avoid buying shoes from a mail-order catalog or the Internet. Even if these sources offer money-back guarantees and free shipping, it doesn't mean you've found a bargain. There is simply no way to assess a shoe's quality, fit, and feel by looking at a picture in a catalog or on a Web site.

Shopping for shoes

Before you purchase any shoes, ask about service and return policies. For example, some retailers may be willing to make low- or no-cost adjustments to the shoes or insoles and allow exchanges or returns. Others may not. A reasonable return policy would allow for a full refund or credit for the return within thirty days of shoes that have not been soiled or damaged. I recommend that you wear new shoes indoors only until you are absolutely certain that you will keep them. It can take a few days to assess how comfortable a shoe is, so make sure the store has a reasonable exchange and return policy. If the store's policy is unreasonable, look elsewhere.

When you go shopping for new shoes, bring a pair or two of your most comfortable shoes along, and be prepared to tell the salesperson as much as possible about what you like and don't like about the shoes. The salesperson can gain valuable clues by evaluating your worn shoes. Wear patterns on the sole reveal how the foot transfers weight. Stretched or creased areas of the upper give clues about the fit. Even the insole or liner in the shoe can reveal pressure points, especially in the ball of the foot.

Before you try on any shoes, the salesperson should take three measurements of your feet, while you are standing:

(1) heel-to-toe length (measured from the heel to the end of the longest toe)

(2) heel-to-ball length (measured from the heel to the large joint of the big toe)

(3) the width at the ball (measured across the large joints of the toes, which is usually the widest point of the foot)

These measurements are only a starting point. The size may have to be adjusted up or down once the shoe can be evaluated on the foot. Some shoe stores may use a computer or pressure mats to assess shape of the foot and how it distributes weight. Some in-store computer systems will even print out a list of suggested shoe models after the foot has been scanned. This information can be useful, but be warned: high-tech computers are no substitute for knowledgeable shoe experts.

Once the measurements are taken, the salesperson can suggest some options for you. A good salesperson will recommend shoes based on your needs, not the stylishness of the shoe. There is an old joke in the shoe industry that the comfort of a shoe is inversely related to its attractiveness, but that doesn't mean that you have to wear ugly shoes in order to be comfortable. The truth is, there are plenty of supportive, foot-friendly shoes that look great.

Shoe shopping should be done at the end of the day when the feet are at their largest due to the natural swelling that occurs as a normal part of activity.

Checking the fit

The fit of a shoe can only be evaluated while you are standing with the shoe on. The heel-to-toe fit is determined by where the longest toe falls within the tip of the shoe. (The longest toe isn't always the big toe; for one out of five people, the second toe is the longer.) Heel-to-toe fit is typically checked by gently compressing the end of the toe box with the fingers or thumb. A properly fitting shoe will have about one-half inch of space between its tip and the end of the longest toe. Most people have one foot that is slightly larger than the other, so

Shoe Wear Patterns

Some people would have you believe that they can tell everything about your feet by looking at the soles of your shoes, much like a fortuneteller looking into a crystal ball. While the pattern of wear on a shoe can reveal some details about your foot and gait, a true foot expert can learn much more by watching you walk without shoes than by looking at your shoe wear pattern. The majority of shoe wear patterns are remarkably similar, even for those with foot problems. In fact, almost all people wear out the outside of the sole's heel. Evaluating the shoe wear pattern can be helpful, but it is just a small part of a thorough evaluation and fitting.

make sure to check both of your feet for length—the larger foot first. Some retailers will split up different shoe sizes to accommodate differences in foot length. Most people, however, do not need two different sizes. If a pair of shoes fits properly in the heel and elsewhere, there will be no problem with the extra toe room in the shoe of the smaller foot. A good fit allows room to wiggle the toes without restriction in both shoes.

The heel-to-ball fit is checked by watching the wearer walk in the shoes. The fitter will look to see that the shoes flex and flare properly at the ball of the foot as the heel is raised. With good-fitting shoes, there is no pinching across the shoe upper and the sole should flex directly under the ball of the foot.

The width is checked by placing the thumb and forefinger across the widest part of the forefoot and squeezing. If the foot is stretching the upper tightly, then the shoe is too narrow—especially if it stretched wider than the sole. If the upper is loose and there is side-to-side movement in the forefoot, then the shoe is too wide. For shoes with

American Shoe Sizing

An increase of one shoe size—for example, from size 7 to size 8—is an increase of about one-third of an inch, primarily in length. A half-size increase, then, is an increase of about one-sixth of an inch. An increase in width size—going from a C to a D width, for example—adds about one-fourth of an inch in width. There is more variability in width sizing than length sizing among manufacturers. From narrowest to widest, the sequence of width sizing is alphabetical and ranges from 5A (or AAAAA) to 6E (or EEEEEE)—a total of fourteen widths. Since most retailers do not have the space to stock all width options, and not all shoes are made in all width options, some manufacturers simply denote the width of the shoe as narrow, medium, or wide, using the letters "N," "M," and "W."

removable insoles, you can check the width by removing the insole and standing on top of it to make sure that your foot is not wider than the footbed of the shoe. Some people are in the habit of wearing shoes a size too long in order to accommodate their width. With more width sizing available today, this is rarely necessary anymore.

Heel fit is important to limit slipping—and blistering as consequence of the slipping. The truest test of heel fit is walking. The heel does not need to be absolutely immobile—a quarter-inch of play is acceptable. But if the heel is slipping noticeably on each step, you should look for another shoe.

The shape of the toe box (the part of the shoe that encloses the toes) is often overlooked by customers—and fitters—during fitting. A toe box that tapers too much can cause problems for those with wider feet. If the little toe feels crowded, a wider shoe or a shoe with a more rounded toe box is recommended.

Collar height should also be considered when fitting shoes. Collar height refers to how high the collar, or rim of the shoe opening, sits on the ankle. Some collars are high and can put pressure on the ankle bones. Women tend to have lower-set ankles than men, so they are more sensitive to pressure from the shoe's collar. If you have ankles that are sensitive or have a tendency to swell, pay attention to how the collar fits around your ankles. Look for shoes with well-padded or low-cut collars.

Take a walk

You can't properly evaluate a pair of shoes if you don't walk in them. So, lace up your prospective new shoes and take a stroll around the store. There's no need to be embarrassed about this. It's expected. Some stores even have treadmills or walking paths. And there's no need to be in a hurry. Wear the shoes for as long as it takes to decide whether they are right for you.

Remember that comfort is subjective. It's okay to ask if the shoes appear to fit, but don't expect the salesperson to be able to determine which pair of shoes is the "best" or most comfortable for you. In the end, you have to decide whether the shoes look and feel right.

After selecting a pair of shoes, write down the models and sizes of other shoes that were strong candidates just in case an exchange is necessary later on or you decide to purchase an additional pair. Then take the new shoes home and expect to spend a few days gradually breaking them in. Avoid wearing the shoes outside until you are sure that you want to keep them, as most shoe stores will not make exchanges or refunds on shoes that have been worn outdoors.

Breaking in shoes

The phrase "breaking in shoes" makes most podiatrists cringe. By far, the biggest cause of foot sores and ulcers is wearing new shoes. This is especially true for those who have swelling, diabetes, circulation disorders, or poor sensitivity in their feet. Breaking in shoes does *not* mean wearing an uncomfortable shoe until it feels good. Shoes should never be purchased unless they feel comfortable after walking in them at the store. A comfortable, well-fitting shoe should then be worn cautiously until you are certain that you have a proper fit. As most of us have learned, a shoe that is comfortable in the store isn't guaranteed to remain comfortable after hours of active use.

Some people believe that good-quality shoes do not need to be broken in because the leather is so soft. There may be some truth to this, but always assume that a new shoe will need at least some cautious breaking in. A new shoe should be worn for the first time at home and for no longer than an hour. You may gradually increase wearing time over several days. Because the feet typically swell a bit throughout the day, you should wear the shoes at different times of the day while breaking them in. Be aware of pressure points, or "hot spots," when wearing the shoes, especially if blisters form. Leather shoes will stretch and give as they are worn, but be alert for areas of tenderness forming on your feet. Stop wearing the shoes immediately if tender areas develop, and return the shoes if tender areas continue to form after short periods of wear. If a blister develops, let it heal before wearing the shoes again.

Breaking in a new pair of shoes isn't just about a pair of shoes adapting to you. It is also about you adapting to the shoes—their different weight, fit, support, and traction. Wearing new shoes can initially cause muscle fatigue and joint pain. But these problems may resolve as the body adapts to the new shoes.

Synthetic materials do not stretch or give like leather, so they are less likely than leather shoes to adapt to your feet.

Optimizing your new shoes

Let's say that you have broken in your new shoes and are very happy with them except for one or two small problems. Not to worry—there are a number of easy yet effective ways to customize shoes. If these suggestions are not sufficient, more sophisticated shoe modifications can be done by a podiatrist or pedorthist.

Simple shoe-lacing patterns

One simple but effective way to adjust the fit of a shoe is by changing the lacing pattern. For example, a shoe that slips in the heel but otherwise fits well can be adjusted by using a crossover lacing pattern. This pattern works well for those who wear heel lifts or insoles, too. People with arthritis may have bony prominences at the tops of their feet. These prominences are easily irritated by pressure from laces. To prevent this irritation, simply avoid lacing the set of eyelets nearest the troublesome spot. If you need a bit more width in the forefoot, try skipping the eyelets closest to the end of the shoes. This will not only help create room for a wider forefoot but for swollen feet and bunions as well.

LACING TECHNIQUES

Conventional Techniques

Diagonal or Chevron   Parallel

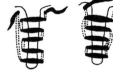

Additional Parallel Techniques

Basic Techniques

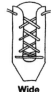

Wide
(For Wide Feet)

Narrow
(For Narrow Feet)

Double Vamp
(Lessens Forefoot Constriction)

Skip Pattern
(Lessens Instep "Pressure Points")

Forefoot Lace
(Lessens Pressure on Great Toe)

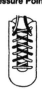

Heel Fit
(Enhances Heel Fit)

High Arch
(Minimizes Pressure on Instep)

Special Techniques

Oxford
(Prevents Loosening of Laces)

Double Knot
(Prevents Laces from Untying)

To make the shoes easier to put on and take off, while still allowing for a secure fit, you can use elastic laces. Elastic laces are inexpensive and let you slip your shoes on and off without having to retie them each time.

If you have arthritis in your hands, poor vision, or some other condition that makes lacing your shoes difficult or impractical, a pedorthist can often convert a lace-up shoe to a shoe with hook-and-loop strap closure.

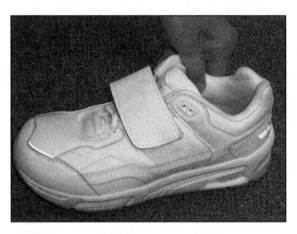

The shape of the laces can affect the feel of the shoe as well. Flat laces stay tied better but do not tighten the shoes as evenly as round laces. Round laces pull more evenly but usually have to be double knotted to stay tied. Elliptical laces combine the qualities of both round and flat laces.

This lace-up shoe has been converted to a hook-and-loop strap closure.

Customizing shoe fit

Some people will require more shoe modification than others—older adults, in particular. By some estimates, up to 25 percent of shoes for older adults should have some type of modification. A good deal of these modifications can be done with padding. Most good shoe stores sell felt pads for customizing the fit of a shoe. Tongue pads can provide extra cushioning over the top of the foot, while keeping the foot from slipping forward in the shoe. Heel pads are adhesive, comma-shaped felt pads that can help secure the heel. You can often find expert advice on padding shoes from stores that have a pedorthist on staff.

Another effective way to customize footwear is the use of insoles and orthotics. In fact, it could be argued that the single most important modification that can be made to improve the support of a shoe is to add one of these devices. The chapter on insoles and orthotics provides detailed information about this topic.

Problems caused by pressure points can sometimes be alleviated by stretching a shoe, though stretching only works with leather shoes. The stretching is done using a ball-and-ring device. Many shoe stores will stretch a shoe for you. Or you can purchase a stretching device at a pharmacy or over the Internet. Stretching shoes works well for relieving pressure points in shoes, but it is not designed or intended to stretch shoes that are too small for the feet.

In some cases, such as severe bunions or hammertoes, cutting the upper with a knife or razor blade may help alleviate foot pain. Make a small, discreet cut directly over a pressure spot or along a seam of the shoe. If necessary, you can patch the inside of the shoe with duct tape or have a shoe repair shop sew in a stretchable fabric or leather patch to prevent debris from getting into the shoe. Though you may feel reluctant to cut into an otherwise perfectly good shoe, this is a viable option for customizing the fit of a shoe.

Difficult-to-fit feet

Those of us who are lucky enough to have feet that fit into conventional-size footwear take for granted that we can find a new pair of shoes quickly with one stop at a good shoe retailer. Those who are less fortunate often dread the thought of having to start a new shoe search. If you have extremely wide, narrow, small, or large feet, you have probably found locating good-fitting shoes to be a frustrating experience. Some consider themselves lucky if a store has any shoes at all in their size. But there is hope for difficult-to-fit feet. More and more manufacturers are adding sizes for wider and larger feet, and more and more retailers are carrying broader ranges of sizes and styles. In addition, manufacturers such as Keen, Saucony and others are making shoes with a "combination" last. These types of lasts offer more width in the forefoot, yet still have a snug-fitting heel. Difficult-to-fit feet are not always about extremes in sizing. Some people simply have very sensitive feet. I have had patients tell me that they have spent three or more hours in a shoe store trying on dozens of different shoes only to leave empty-handed. A possible option in such cases is a custom orthotic that can be moved from shoe to shoe.

Shoes as therapy

If you are currently dealing with a foot injury or have a history of chronic foot pain, you need to remember that footwear is often a crucial component of your therapy. Your feet cannot heal if your shoes do not protect them. And, if your shoes are contributing to your foot pain, you should not realistically expect your pain to resolve until you make a change to a different type of footwear.

Sometimes, making footwear changes means wearing only your most confortable and supportive shoes until your pain resolves. For example, if you are vulnerable to plantar fasciitis, you will want to wear shoes that can accommodate an insole and only gradually increase the time you wear other shoes *after* the pain has improved. Sometimes, footwear changes involve eliminating, permanently, shoes that cause pain. Through trail and error, you will become an expert on how and when you need to wear certain shoes to keep your feet feeling their best.

Shoe do's and don'ts

The following section summarizes some of the most important points of this chapter. It is based on my experiences both as a podiatrist and a shoe store salesperson.

Shoe do's

- Splurge on at least one pair of good shoes from a reputable retailer. You'll have to spend about one hundred dollars for a good pair, but it's money well spent. (Note, however, that higher prices don't always mean higher quality.) Discount retailers may offer bargains, but if the shoes are of poor quality, you aren't sized properly, or you aren't offered good advice, your bargain shoes will just end up in the closet next to your other uncomfortable shoes. A properly fitting, supportive shoe bought with the guidance of an expert shoe retailer or pedorthist is worth every penny.

- Shop later in the day. Feet tend to swell over the course of the day, so you want to make sure to accommodate for this change when having your feet fit. Don't worry, the shoe isn't going to be "sloppy" before your foot swells if it is fit properly. Think of a sandal when evaluating the fit—a sandal with a nice strap across the instep, a snug heel strap, and plenty of wiggle room for your toes. The shoe should only be snug in the back two-thirds, from the heel through the arch, with enough width to accommodate the ball of the foot and a rounded toe box to prevent the toes from being squeezed together. By hugging the instep and heel, a good shoe will fit well early in the day and retain that fit throughout the day, with enough room in the forefoot to allow for some normal swelling.

- Buy running shoes for walking and all-around wear. Running shoes have the best combination of cushioning, stability, support, and breathability. You don't have to be a runner to appreciate and enjoy good running shoes. In fact, 70 percent of the running shoes sold aren't used for running at all but for walking.

- If two different models feel good to you, put one model on your left foot and the other model on your right, comparing them foot to foot as you stroll around the store.

- Wear your newly purchased shoes (with socks) around the house for a few days before venturing outdoors. If there are any problems with the shoes, you'll get no hassles when you return them.

- Minimize the amount of time you wear uncomfortable shoes. Even wearing athletic shoes to and from work or a social function can help minimize some of the pain you might feel later.

- Replace or repair your shoes when they show signs of wear. A worn-out heel will alter how your foot distributes pressure, stressing the bones, muscles, and connective tissue; a stretched or torn upper robs you of support, increasing your risk of rolling off the shoe and spraining an ankle or falling.

Shoe don'ts

- Don't expect that just because you bought brand-name shoes or spent a lot of money for pair of shoes that they will be good for your feet. Finding the proper shoe is only partly about brand and price point.

- Don't assume that more cushioning will solve your foot problems. Excessively soft shoes actually put more strain on the feet and legs. The best shoes offer a balanced combination of cushioning, support, and stability.

- Don't expect to find good support and good fit in dress shoes. Few dress shoes—and this is especially the case with high heels—offer truly healthy support and fit. This doesn't mean you should never wear dress shoes, but you should minimize their use.

- Don't focus on shoe size. There is no such thing as an absolute size 7—or an absolute size anything—when it comes to shoes. There are great variations in sizes, even within the same brand. The size you are measured at is only a ballpark figure, a starting point. The only true way to gauge shoe size is to put a shoe on your foot. Is there adequate room for your toes in that size 7? If not, try size 7-1/2 or larger.

- Don't expect your foot pain to improve if you insist on buying the same types of shoes and shoe sizes that you've bought in the past. Studies show that improperly fitting shoes are the most significant contributing factor in chronic foot problems. Your feet won't feel better until you truly change your shoes.

- Don't forget about width. It's easier today than ever before to find shoes in widths that fit you. Many brands are now offering a variety of widths in popular models. Like shoe sizes, widths can vary widely even within the same brand. Keep trying until you find the right width for you. The benefits are worth it, especially for those with swollen feet, nerve problems, and bunions.

- Don't buy your shoes from a catalog or off the Internet unless you are buying the exact same model in the exact same size of a shoe you already own or have previously been fitted for the shoes you are buying. There is simply no substitute for trying a shoe on, being properly fitted, asking questions, and comparing a number of different brands and models.

- Don't expect a new shoe to completely and magically solve your foot problems. Most foot problems take time to resolve, and a good shoe may be only one piece of the treatment puzzle. You may still need the guidance of your doctor and other types of treatment.

- Don't strangle your feet by tying the laces too tight. Your feet have tendons, nerves, and blood vessels on at their tops that can be compressed by laces that are too tight. The laces should be just snug enough to keep the shoes from slipping. There are lacing patterns that can snug up the shoe without creating pressure. Or a tongue pad can be placed on the tongue of the shoe to snug up the midfoot without the need for over-tightening the laces.

- Don't wear slippers if you have foot pain or poor balance. Slippers provide no support or cushioning, tend to fit poorly, and wear out quickly. Some studies have linked slippers to falls and increased foot pain. More protective footwear is recommended.

Foot problems and shoe solutions

Foot pain can often be effectively addressed simply be selecting a more appropriate shoe. In fact, there are specific shoe features that can help to alleviate most sources of foot pain. Many of the shoe suggestions listed below work even better when combined with the protective products and techniques discussed in the chapters on specific foot conditions.

Problem: Corns on the tops of toes

Solution: If you have both hammertoes and corns, look for a shoe with extra depth and a rounded toe box. (A rounded shoe toe box is the ideal shape for any wearer.)

Problem: Corns on the sides or between toes

Solution: Shoes that are sized properly in width and offer a rounded toe box will decrease the side-to-side pressure that often contributes to these types of painful calluses. Corns on the smallest toe are often caused by rotation of the toe, so padding the toe with a gel sleeve in addition to wearing wider shoes often helps alleviate this problem.

Problem: Bunions

Solution: Choose a shoe with a wide forefoot. For larger bunions, you may also need to have the shoe's pressure points stretched. In addition, good arch support and a toe spacer can decrease the workload on the big toe joint and pressure on the bunion, decreasing pain.

Problem: Sweaty feet or athlete's foot

Solution: Look for shoes that have a mesh upper. These shoes offer optimal breathability. Solid leather and synthetic uppers don't breathe as well as mesh cloth (natural or synthetic). Consider wearing sandals They also work well to alleviate sweaty feet and aid the treatment of athlete's foot. In addition, synthetic wicking socks keep the feet drier than cotton socks. The addition of cooling, moisture-absorbent powders are a good complement to these footwear.

Problem: Pinched nerve or neuroma

Solution: Look for shoes that have a wide forefoot and rounded toe box. This will decrease the pressure on the affected nerve. Often, you may also benefit from a metatarsal pad or orthotics inside the shoe. Avoid wearing high-heeled shoes.

Problem: Poor balance or frequent falls

Solution: Shoes that keep your feet close to the ground (flats) will help you maintain better balance. Elevated or high heels, as well as poorly fitting shoes, will increase your risk of falling. Avoid thick, cushioned shoes, looking instead for shoes that offer support and stability and have thin midsoles and moderate amounts of cushioning.

Problem: Difficulty tying laces or excessive pain caused by laces

Solution: There are a good number of slip-on shoes and sandals that can help you overcome difficulty or pain associated with lacing up shoes. Most manufacturers also make shoes with Velcro closures instead of laces, and many shoe repair shops can convert lace-up closures to Velcro closures. For those who experience pain but want to keep lacing their shoes, consider elastic laces that secure the shoe while reducing pressure on trouble spots.

Problem: Fallen arches or flat feet

Solution: Look for straight-lasted shoes with a stability device such as a medial post. (For more information, see the section on shoe construction earlier in this chapter.) These features will support your foot well and also accommodate additional orthotics.

Problem: Arthritis in the midfoot or top of the arch

Solution: A semistraight- or straight-lasted shoe with a medial post provides support and helps transfer weight from the heel to the forefoot. Firm orthotics can enhance the support of the shoe as well. Lacing patterns can be changed in order to decrease pressure on the top of the arches. A pedorthist can add devices to the shoes sole to protect arthritic joints in the midfoot.

Problem: Arthritis of the big toe joint

Solution: A shoe that is stiff at the ball of the foot and has a medial post will help protect the joint, as well as accommodate additional orthotics. Sometimes stretching the shoe upper at the joint site can relieve pressure on bony protrusions that develop with this type of arthritis. For more severe cases, a metatarsal bar or a rocker bottom can be added to the shoe by a certified pedorthist or shoe repair shop.

Problem: Numb feet

Solution: Look for shoes with cloth linings, soft leather uppers, rounded toe boxes, and semistraight lasts. Break your new shoes in gradually and cautiously. Check your feet regularly and often. The most likely time to develop foot sores or infections occurs when breaking in shoes.

Problem: Ingrown toenails

Solution: In addition to good nail care, make sure your shoes have at least a half-inch of space between the end of the shoe and your longest toe. Look for shoes with a rounded toe box to decrease pressure on the nail. Also, consider wearing sandals whenever you can. Toe spacers can help if changes in the alignment of the toes are contributing to the problem.

Problem: Plantar fasciitis (or pain on the bottom of the heel)

Solution: Look for shoes that support the arch well. In general, running shoes are best, especially those that have a medial post or other motion-control feature. Remember, shoes that are too soft can actually make heel pain worse. Often, you'll have to add supportive insoles to the shoes as well.

Problem: Haglund's bump, Achilles tendonitis (or pain to the back of the heel)

Solution: Decreasing pressure on the painful area can be done with open-back footwear such as clogs or sandals. In some cases, a slight elevation to the heel can take tension off the tendon where it attaches to the heel. Heel sleeves, pads, or cups can be added to the shoes to relieve pressure on the heel as well.

Problem: Ankle pain

Solution: Shoes with maximum stability will decrease the strain on the ankle joint and provide a firm platform for supportive insoles and ankle braces if necessary. Running shoes with a straight or semistraight lasts and medial posts work can provide relief, as can casual shoes with a thin midsole, which keep the feet close to the ground, maximizing stability.

Problem: Heel slipping

Solution: Do not buy narrow shoes just because your heel is slipping. You will do so to the detriment of the rest of your foot. Fit the forefoot first, and then address any heel slippage by lacing the shoes differently or adding heel pads to the shoe to snug up the heel cup. If necessary, try another model or brand. Don't be overly concerned with heel movement. Your heel is not supposed to be locked in the shoe; a certain amount of play is normal and desirable. If the shoes do not cause pain or blisters on your heel, then there is no reason to make any change.

Socks

Socks are an important part of footwear. Socks protect the skin from friction. Socks keep the feet dry, minimizing bacteria and fungus. Those who wear clean socks will have less foot odor and their shoes will last longer because the socks protect the shoe from the oils and moisture of the feet.

The most common reason I hear from patients for not wearing socks is that they are too difficult to get on. A device called a sock donner can make this task much easier. This tube-like device stretches the sock and helps pull it up the leg with less strain on the hands or back.

Despite commonly accepted beliefs, cotton socks are not the best choice for good footcare. Natural wool and synthetic fabrics such as nylon are better at wicking moisture from the feet than cotton. When cotton gets damp from sweat, it retains the moisture and keeps it close to the skin. This increases the risk of blisters, athlete's foot, and general discomfort. Synthetic fabrics and wool pull the moisture away from the skin, which cools the feet and minimizes moisture-related problems.

Sock "innovations" are becoming more common in recent years. Some socks are touted as having extra-thick fabric padding on the soles to provide more cushioning, or elastic bands in the arch to provide support. These claims are exaggerated. The amount of padding or support provided by the sock is insignificant. Insoles and shoes provide the most durable forms of cushioning and support. Buying socks for the quality of the fabric is more important than buying for cushioning or arch support.

Some socks are capable of providing support to the lower legs and ankles to minimize swelling. Compression stockings are snug stockings that are designed to maintain a supportive pressure around the legs. This pressure helps the veins return blood to the heart, which decreases the amount of swelling that occurs in the lower legs. Commercially available compression stockings can be found in most pharmacies and work well for mild swelling. Prescription compression stockings are ordered by physicians and are custom fit by a technician. They are indicated for chronic swelling and peripheral vascular diseases.

Compression stockings can also decrease the risk for developing blood clots. A common risk factor for developing a deep vein thrombosis is being immobile for extended periods of time. Those who travel frequently should consider wearing compression stockings.

Understanding shoes and their effect on the health of the feet is the first step in making informed choices when selecting footwear. The huge number of different shoe styles on the market can be overwhelming and confusing. But if you take your time to learn what footwear features work best for your unique needs, you will be better able to sort through the perplexing options available to you.

Seek out quality shoe retailers and medical professionals and expect to make use of some of the shoe products and modification techniques that can make a good shoe even better for you. The next chapter will discuss insoles and orthotics, which provide the best options for truly customizing footwear.

9

Insoles and Orthotics

In the last few years, the number of foot comfort products on the market has exploded. With the increased availability of such products has come increased confusion among consumers. How do you know which products you need? How do you know which products are effective? As discussed throughout this book, wearing footwear and footwear accessories that support the feet properly is often the best way to address common foot problems. Unfortunately, there a number of shoes and shoe products that do very little to support the foot. And there are expensive "custom" devices that are little more than overpriced arch supports with greatly exaggerated claims about their benefits. Finding the right product for a particular condition or problem can be a frustrating, costly, and time-consuming process. This chapter provides information that I hope will make this process a little less difficult.

An insole or orthotic is only as supportive as the shoe in which it is placed. Shoes that do not have room for an insole or orthotic are not capable of helping a painful foot, and unsupportive shoes will not magically become supportive by adding an insole or orthotic.

Seek out footcare specialists

Sometimes it seems as if everyone is selling insoles and orthotics. Web sites, infomercials, mail-order catalogs, discount store

Cushioning alone is rarely the answer to foot pain. Just as important, if not more so, is support to maintain the proper alignment of the foot and ankle joints. Firm support helps the feet and body absorb step impact. Excessive cushioning, on the other hand, makes it harder for the feet to absorb impact because, as the cushioning compresses, the joints fall out of alignment. Excessive cushioning can also increase strain on muscles and tendons, while dulling sensation and compromising balance.

pharmacies, and pseudo-medical "clinics" are just some of the places that insoles and orthotics are offered for sale. The recognized authorities on insoles and orthotics, however, are podiatrists and certified pedorthists. In addition, some orthopedists and physical therapitst subspecialize in the feet and ankles. These are the experts you should see if you need relief for a foot problem.

A podiatrist or orthopedist can do a thorough evaluation of your feet and make detailed recommendations for treating any problems you may have—from simple shoe changes to surgery. Unlike podiatrists and orthopedists, pedorthists and physical therapists are not trained to diagnose foot conditions; but they are qualified to make and implement treatment plans using insoles and orthotics once a diagnosis has been made.

Medical professionals may recommend any of many different types of insert devices to treat a particular foot problem. These insert devices are manufactured under a number of labels, including "foot beds," "arch supports," "insoles," "orthotics," and "shoe inserts." In this chapter, the term *insoles* will be used to refer to over-the-counter inserts, and the term *orthotics* will be used to describe doctor-prescribed, custom-made devices. Shoe-padding devices such as heel cups, arch supports, and metatarsal pads will be discussed separately at the end of the chapter.

What are insoles?

Insoles are prefabricated, store-bought inserts that add support or cushioning to shoes. Choosing the right insole for you depends on many factors, including your foot type, the style of the shoe, the type of activity you plan to use the shoe for, and the condition of your foot. Even your weight affects which type of insole might be best for you. Insoles can be found at pharmacies, Internet sites, shoe stores, sporting goods stores, and footcare retailers.

Most insoles are made of foam, silicone gel, rubber, or plastic. They may be soft to cushion and distribute pressure, or they may be firm to provide sturdy arch support. Some can be customized by heating and forming them to the foot. Many can be modified with pads or other devices by podiatrists or pedorthists. Insoles are always sold in pairs and should be worn as a pair—even when treating only one painful foot. Using only one insole can create strain on the knees, hips, or back.

If a soft, cushioned insole has failed to relieve foot pain, then seek out a firmer, more supportive device and not a softer one. Often, a firm insole is more effective at supporting the foot and relieving pressure.

What are orthotics?

Orthotics are custom-made supportive devices for the feet, prescribed by a medical professional to treat a specific foot or leg condition. There are two types of orthotics: functional and accommodative:

(1) **Functional orthotics** are used to treat the foot problems of active people. Functional orthotics are designed to improve the function of the feet by realigning the joints and correcting biomechanical problems.

(2) **Accommodative orthotics** are designed to accommodate foot deformities or to evenly distribute step pressure for patients with numbness in the feet or risk factors for skin injury. Patients with diabetes, peripheral vascular disease, or a history of foot ulcers benefit from soft, conforming, accommodative orthotics.

Customized orthotics offer a higher level of precision, support, function, and effectiveness than over-the-counter insoles. After a thorough exam that may include gait analysis and, if appropriate, X-rays of the feet and lower legs, the feet are cast in plaster or foam, or are digitally scanned with a computer to map their shape and contour. An orthotics lab then manufactures the needed orthotics with medical-grade materials using either the cast or scan and the podiatrist's prescription.

Why would I need shoe inserts?

Shoe inserts such as insoles and orthotics are used to treat specific foot problems—heel pain, arch pain, aching feet, arthritis, and other complaints. There are quite a few foot and lower-leg conditions commonly treated using inserts. These conditions include:

- arthritis
- bunions
- foot conditions related to diabetes
- flat feet
- foot ulcers
- hallux limitus/rigidus
- heel spurs
- metatarsalgia
- neuroma
- peripheral neuropathy (numbness)
- plantar fasciitis
- sports injuries
- surgically repaired feet/ankles/legs
- tendonitis
- weak ankles

The benefits of properly selected and fitted insoles and orthotics are undeniable and often dramatic. It should be noted, however, that inserts typically do not "cure" foot conditions but rather treat them by relieving one or more symptoms and preventing conditions from getting worse. Correct use of insoles and orthotics can:

- decrease foot pain
- decrease the risk of falling
- decrease fatigue in the legs and lower back
- distribute pressure
- improve balance
- improve shoe comfort
- prevent calluses
- protect arthritic joints
- support collapsing arches.

Insoles

Insoles work best with shoes that come with removable insoles. Conversely, there are many kinds of shoes that will not work well with insoles. Open-back shoes, high heels and many kinds of dress shoes, cowboy boots, and extremely tight shoes do not accommodate insoles well—or orthotics, for that matter. Neither do most sandals work well with insoles or orthotics. However, some sandals are specifically designed to accommodate inserts—Naot and Finn Comfort, for example. And brands such as Rockport, Ecco and Munro make dress shoes with removable insoles.

A good test of any insole is the pinch test. Place the insole between the thumb and forefinger. If it can be pinched flat with the fingers, then the insole is neither thick nor dense enough to provide therapeutic cushioning.

Shoes with removable insoles

The benefits of removable insoles are two-fold: the removable insoles that come with the shoes can be modified if necessary to treat certain foot problems, or they can be replaced with a more supportive insole or customized insole or orthotic.

Over-the-counter insoles

The best insoles range in price from fifteen to fifty dollars. Insoles costing less than fifteen dollars are usually not as supportive or durable as more expensive insoles and rarely offer much benefit for the feet. Insoles costing more than fifty dollars are not usually worth the extra expense. They may even be inferior in quality to mid-priced insoles. (In some cases, a quality custom device can be made for less than an overpriced commercial insole.)

Drug stores and large chain discount retailers tend to offer lower-priced insoles, ranging in price from eight to twenty dollars. Shoe stores and sporting goods stores usually sell the better, mid-priced insoles, costing from fifteen to sixty dollars. The best products come in packages that allow the buyer to stand on the insole to feel its support. The brand Superfeet offers sample sizes that can be slipped into shoes. Again, just as for buying shoes, I highly recommend trying insoles on before buying them.

The more brands and models of insoles a retailer offers, the more likely that retailer will have a product that is comfortable and useful for your feet. You wouldn't buy shoes from a store that offered only one or two models of shoes, so don't settle for any insole if you haven't had an opportunity to compare it to other brands. As with shoes, you can't tell which insole is going to be most comfortable for you until you've tried a number of different ones on.

Be cautious of any insole that is "guaranteed" to work. No single treatment or device works for every patient 100 percent of the time. As popular wisdom warns, if it sounds too good to be true, then it probably is. Honest, experienced professionals who sell insoles or make orthotics know that every patient is unique and not every product will work for every foot.

Insoles (and orthotics) can add significantly to shoe comfort, but they cannot magically change an unsupportive shoe into a supportive one. The better insoles will take up more room, so not all shoes can accommodate them. Sometimes, it may be necessary to purchase shoes a half size larger to accommodate supportive insoles. Dress shoes tend to be especially difficult to fit with insoles. Even in those cases where it is possible to fit dress shoes with insoles, the shoe are too often simply a bad fit—with or without insoles.

Soft insoles versus firm insoles

Most people with foot pain will seek more cushioning for their feet either by buying a softer shoe or adding a soft insole to an existing shoe. The problem with cushioning is that it comes at a cost. When something soft is placed between the feet and the ground, the feet become unstable, causing the joints to fall out of alignment, which leads to more impact on—and more stress fatigue in—the joints, bones, and muscles.

You don't have to wear insoles all day, every day. Wear them only as needed to maintain comfort and minimize foot pain. This may mean restricting their use to certain activities or times of day.

Soft, foam insoles are usually the lowest-priced insoles, which makes them appealing to consumers. Unfortunately, you tend to get what you pay for. Most foam insoles are too thin and flimsy to offer much support—or real cushioning. (Thin gel insoles work better than foam, but, again, are often too thin to be effective, especially for more serious cases of foot pain.)

Soft insoles made from rubbery materials or silicone gels have become extremely popular in recent last years. Television advertisements proclaim the near ecstatic cushioning benefits of the insoles. While these soft insoles can provide some cushioning and relief from pressure-related pain, they typically do not have enough support to offer protection from arthritis, plantar fasciitis, or collapsing arches. Among the better soft insoles are products made by New Balance, Spenco, Sorbathane, and Dr. Scholl's.

Firm insoles or insoles that combine a firm arch support with cushioned cover material can benefit a number of foot conditions. Most people benefit from a firm insole with moderate cushioning, but this is especially true for active people. The firm part of these insoles is typically made from plastic, fiberglass, or dense foam. The firm part helps maintain alignment in the rearfoot and arch. Firm insoles have added benefits in that they tend to last longer and are easier to customize than softer inserts. Recommended brands of firm insoles include Superfeet, Tacco (if a compromise is needed for dress shoes), Birkenstock, Power Step, and Spenco. Keep in mind that some of these brands make many different models of insoles. For example, Spenco makes both soft and firm insoles.

Once insoles have been purchased, it can take a few days for the body to adapt to the additional support. It is not unusual to experience temporary aches or fatigue in the feet or legs after inserting the insole. Start by wearing the insoles for only a few hours a day and gradually increase your wear time. Foot problems don't develop overnight, so don't expect them to disappear overnight.

You may find it beneficial to wear firm insoles with a pair of shoes that offer maximum support until your pain resolves. Foot pain resolves much more quickly if the foot is supported well and consistently. Once the pain has resolved, many people can return to wearing less supportive shoes, but be warned that wearing bad shoes will only cause the pain to recur. Periodic use of the insoles and supportive shoes may be necessary to treat flare-ups. Often, when an insole works well, people prefer to wear it just for comfort.

Short and full-length insoles

Insoles come in many different shapes and sizes. Shorter insoles, extending from the heel to just before the ball of the foot, control the heel and arch but do not provide much support for the forefoot. They are used for treating heel and arch pain. Full-length insoles extend from the heel to the toes. They work as well as short insoles for heel and arch pain, but are more versatile for treating pain in the forefoot and ball of the foot. Full-length insoles fit better in shoes that have a removable insole and are the preferred insole for athletic shoes.

Dress shoe insoles

As mentioned above, dress shoes accommodate insoles less well than other types of shoes. However, thin, low-profile insoles, while not as supportive as other devices, can provide some support for those who need to wear dress shoes regularly. Tacco and Superfeet both make dress shoe insoles, and Insolia is an insole made especially for women's high-heeled shoes.

Odor-reducing and antibacterial insoles

Some insoles are designed to decrease foot odor. Many contain activated charcoal that absorbs odors. More recently developed insoles contain antibacterials, including silver and copper, to control the buildup of odor-causing bacteria and fungus. These types of insoles are effective for those whose feet are prone to sweating and odor, especially when combined with good hygiene, proper sock selection, and the use of foot powders.

Magnetic insoles

Not long ago, magnetic bracelets, necklaces, belts, and even insoles were widely available. And there seems to be a revival of interest in the healing power of magnets every few years. However, scientific research has not shown any benefits from using magnets to treat medical conditions. Stick with supportive—nonmagnetic—insoles to treat your foot condition. We know they work.

Heat-moldable insoles

Some manufacturers offer insoles that can be heated and then shaped to the feet. These types of insoles can increase comfort, but should not be used to treat an injury without visiting a podiatrist or pedorthist first. Molding insoles to the feet can cause more problems than they solve if not fitted properly. These types of insoles are usually more expensive than other insoles and require a high level of knowledge and expertise to modify properly. Some podiatrists and pedorthists dispense a low-cost, "semi-customized" heat-moldable insole that they will mold to your feet for you. This can be a good alternative for those who do not want custom orhotics but have failed to find relief with conventional insoles.

Modifying over-the-counter insoles

Very simple modifications can increase the comfort of an insole and save the cost of a custom device (which may not be covered by insurance). Adding more arch support, for example, can help prevent pain from plantar fasciitis and arthritis. Adding a metatarsal pad can decrease pressure and pain at the ball of the foot. Even painful calluses can be protected with a well-positioned pad.

The best material for modifying an insole is moleskin. Moleskin is an adhesive padding made of cotton or synthetic fiber. It is available in most pharmacies and through the Internet. Moleskin can be cut to any shape and is durable enough to last weeks or even months. Medical-grade moleskin is made from wool. Although it is costs more than standard moleskin, it is more durable than synthetics or cotton.

One of the benefits of better-quality insoles is their versatility and the ease with which they can be modified. Some insoles lend themselves to modification much better than others. Soft insoles that compress easily are extremely difficult to modify because adhesive pads will not stick well to the shifting surface. Firm insoles provide a more durable surface for modifying with pads.

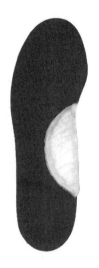

Adding an adhesive moleskin arch pad to an insole can increase comfort and decrease heel and arch pain.

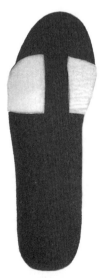

Pressure can be distributed around a painful forefoot callus or bone with a moleskin modification.

Modifications to treat heel pain

Sometimes an insole alone isn't enough to relieve heel pain. Modifications to the insole are needed. For example, increasing the arch support of the insole can decrease pressure on the bottom of the heel by effectively transferring weight from the heel to the forefoot with each step. Arch support also helps prevent the arch from collapsing, which can reduce strain on the plantar fascia. Additional heel cushioning can be added to an insole as well with adhesive heel cushions.

Modifications to treat arch pain

Insole modifications for arch pain may require not only an arch pad but also support under the heel or forefoot. By wedging the feet to prevent excessive collapsing of the arch, the workload on the bones of the arch is decreased. A podiatrist or certified pedorthist should be consulted for this type of insole modification.

Modifications to treat forefoot pain

Forefoot pain is commonly caused by bony prominences, hammertoes, calluses, arthritis, metatarsalgia, or neuromas. Insoles should be modified to address the specific cause or causes of the forefoot pain. Adding arch support can help with many cases of forefoot pain by helping the foot transfer weight more efficiently and evenly. Other modifications are aimed at decreasing pressure on painful areas.

Metatarsal pads are felt adhesive pads shaped like teardrops. They can be placed on the top of an insole at the end of the arch to decrease pressure on the ball of the foot. These pads work well to treat a number of sources of forefoot pain, particularly metatarsalgia, neuromas, and calluses on the bottom of the feet. There are many over-the-counter pads that claim to be "metatarsal pads," but most podiatrists and pedorthists use the wool-felt pads made by medical companies such as Hapad. Most people instinctively want to place the pad under the ball of the foot, but this should be avoided. A properly placed metatarsal pad will feel as though it is supporting the end of the arch instead of the ball of the foot.

Pressure-relief pads, or aperture pads, distribute pressure away from a bony prominences. They sometimes need to be used in combination with a metatarsal pad. The most effective way to alleviate the pain caused by a bony prominence is to place padding around, rather than directly on, the affected area. This can be done by cutting a piece of moleskin to the size and shape needed. For example, donut- or horseshoe-shaped pads placed around an area of pain work well to remove pressure. Or, a "channel" effect can be created by placing parallel strips of moleskin on either side of a painful area. Because the padding compresses over time, it may have to be replaced or reinforced every few weeks. The pads will last longer if placed under the insole instead of on top of it.

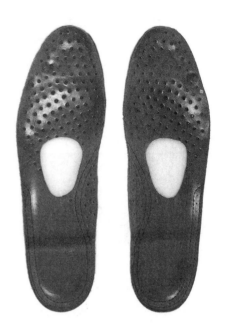

Metatarsal pads have been added directly to the shoes' removable insoles to treat forefoot pain.

Orthotics

Orthotics are sometimes needed for foot conditions that do not respond to over-the-counter insoles or for foot types that simply need a higher level of control. Orthotics differ from over-the-counter insoles in that they are doctor-prescribed, custom-made, and manufactured from medical-grade materials. To prescribe and construct an orthotic device properly, a podiatrist or orthopedist needs to perform a thorough physical exam and gait evaluation. Periodic adjustments or alterations may also be necessary. Orthotics are generally more durable than insoles, lasting up to three years or longer.

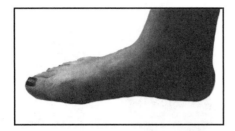

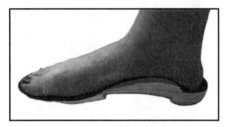

A collapsing arch (top) supported by a custom orthotic (below).

Custom orthotics must be made by a foot specialist. Orthotics should never be purchased at health fairs, through the mail, off the Internet, or from any source other than a licensed foot specialist. Unscrupulous sellers of orthotics will make exaggerated claims about the benefits of their devices and often disparage medically prescribed orthotics. Only podiatrists and medical doctors can diagnose foot problems. And general practitioners will refer patients to podiatrists if there is an indication that orthotics may be needed.

One benefit of getting your orthotics through a licensed foot specialist is that he or she can help you determine if the device is covered by your health insurance. Some health insurance plans will pay for one pair of orthotics per year, others may only cover one every three years. Medicare covers the cost of orthotics for only a limited number of foot conditions and injuries. Find out what your insurance plan covers before having any orthotics created. Even if orthotics are not covered by health insurance, they may still be worth the investment. Many clinics are happy to offer payment plans or varying levels of customized or "semicustomized" devices for those on a budget. Insurance coverage for orthotic devices is highly variable and always changing, but one thing is certain: insurance companies will not reimburse you for any orthotics you purchase from unlicensed vendors.

Make sure that the podiatrist, pedorthist, or clinic you are working with provides follow-up care and orthotics service after they have been prescribed. Even though orthotics are custom made, they can still require adjustment or alteration to work well or to meet changing needs.

Other foot support devices

Insoles and orthotics will support and protect your feet better than other types of devices. However, some foot conditions may not require the support that orthotics offer, and not all shoes are versatile enough to accommodate an insole. Lower-profile shoe inserts can provide minimal or temporary support when insoles or orthotics either aren't necessary or can't be worn. A simple arch support or heel cup can be better than no support at all. The devices described below can be found in most pharmacies and shoe stores.

Heel cups

Heel cups, or heel pads, are cushioned pads that fit easily into shoes at the heel. They are usually made from silicone gel, rubber, or foam. They help relieve the pain caused by pressure from heel spurs and plantar fasciitis. If the cushioning of the heel cups fails to relieve pain after one week of use, then an insole that supports the arch may be necessary.

Arch supports

The term "arch supports" has multiple meanings. In the strictest sense, arch supports are crescent-shaped devices for filling in the area under the arch of the foot. Arch supports do not provide as much protection as insoles, but they can be effective in relieving arch pain and occasionally heel pain. Tacco makes a firm leather arch support that can placed in shoes with adhesive. Moleskin can be cut and stacked to serve as an arch support as well.

An arch support has been added to the shoe on the right.

Heel lifts

Heel lifts are prescribed to correct inequalities in limb length and to treat Achilles tendonitis. Some so-called heel lifts are so spongy and compress so much that they provide no lift at all. The best heel lifts are made from rubber or other firm materials. Heel lifts should be used in both shoes if treating Achilles tendonitis, but in only one shoe if treating an inequality in limb length. Adjust-A-Lift makes a heel lift with three one-eighth-inch layers of thick rubber, each of which can be removed as needed to achieve the most comfortable level of elevation. If you suspect that one of your legs may be longer than the other, I would recommend that you see a medical professional before attempting to treat yourself.

Gel heel sleeves

A heel sleeve is s sock-like cushioned sleeve that slips over the heel to cushion painful heel spurs, heel bumps, or inflamed Achilles tendons. The sleeve has a gel pad at the back of the heel to protect the affected area.

10

Staying Active

Movement is life and without movement life is unthinkable.
—Moshe Fledenkrais

Try to think of a fitness activity that doesn't require healthy feet. Swimming? Rowing? Perhaps. But healthy feet contribute even to these activities—by helping the swimmer maintain balance and by providing the rower with leverage. The feet are the platform for most activities, whether we're standing on them or not.

Being able to move about easily can contribute significantly to your quality of life and emotional well-being. If you are lucky enough to have few limitations on your physical activity, don't take your health for granted. Preserve your good health by exercising regularly. If you do have some physical limitations, you should still try to find ways to be active. Physical activity not only lowers your risk of getting a disease or being injured but also helps you better manage a disease and recover more quickly from an injury.

Researchers who study aging populations have found that those who are physically active are happier, more social, have fewer medical problems, are hospitalized less often, take fewer medications, and live independently for longer periods of time than those who are sedentary.[23] To achieve the benefits of exercise, regular fitness

Benefits of Exercise

Immediate	Long-term
elevated mood	improved balance
reduced stress	stronger muscles and bones
better sleep	greater endurance
improved cardiovascular function	longer life and higher quality of life
lower cholesterol	better able to live independently
lower blood sugar	reduced risk of heart disease, diabetes, high blood pressure, and some cancers
more social interaction	

routines must be maintained. You can lose the benefits of exercise if you abandon your fitness routine.[24] Fortunately, it's never too late to start exercising. You can reverse many of the effects of a sedentary lifestyle at almost any age.[25]

People used to think that they didn't need to exercise as much as they aged. Many even believed that the stress of exercise could worsen diseases such as arthritis and heart disease. We now know that the benefits of regular exercise far outweigh any risks. In fact, your overall health is much more at risk from a sedentary lifestyle than an active one. The incidence of heart disease, diabetes, obesity, hypertension, cancer, and osteoporosis are all higher in those who are sedentary.

The U.S. Surgeon General recommends twenty to thirty minutes of moderate-intensity exercise most days of the week. But 60 percent of Americans do not do even this modest amount of physical activity.[26]

Being physically active is important not only for strength and endurance, but for counteracting the age-related deterioration of normal physical function. As we age, we lose muscle mass and nerve function. This compromises balance and increases the risk of falling. Regular exercise helps maintain muscle strength and nerve function, thereby improving balance and decreasing the risk of falling . Physical decline is rapid with inactivity, so it is important to make physical activity a consistent part of your healthy lifestyle.

Always consult a physician before beginning any exercise program.

Exercise and the older athlete

Older adults are increasingly coming to clinics with injuries sustained while playing sports. While this might sound alarming, it is actually a consequence of a very positive trend. Americans are participating in athletic activities much longer than they used to. Athletes and fitness advocates are continuing to pursue the activities they love despite their age, and many older adults are taking up sports for the first time. It is no longer rare to see retirement-age runners participating in their first marathon. Triathlon competitors in their seventies are beating people half their age. Senior hockey, baseball, and tennis leagues are enjoying record participation. Even adventure sports such as mountain climbing and skydiving are seeing rising participation by older adults.

By far, the most popular form of exercise for older adults is also one of the best forms of exercise: walking. According to American Sports Data Inc., 10.9 million Americans, 55 and older, walked for exercise at least once during 2003. The appeal of walking is obvious: it doesn't require special training, facilities, or equipment; it can be done almost anytime, anywhere; it's cheap; almost anyone can do it; and it's not particularly strenuous or risky.

As I mentioned earlier, the benefits of being physically active far outweigh any risks. These benefits are both immediate and long term. Believe it or not, once you've begun to experience the benefits of exercise, you will actually start to look forward to your workouts. You have to maintain realistic expectations, though. Some of the benefits take time and require consistent effort. While you may not lose a lot of weight or feel like Superman after your first week of exercise, you should find yourself feeling and sleeping better.

That said, expect to experience some fatigue, aches, or energy loss as your body adapts to the stress of increased physical activity. Pace yourself, and hang in there. If it is too difficult to walk for twenty minutes at first, then take two ten-minute walks instead. Allowing your body to recover completely from each workout can be as important as the workout itself. Over time, gradually increase the length of each activity and the number of workouts you are doing. This is the best way to prevent injury and keep yourself from burning out.

It isn't always easy to stay motivated. Even world class athletes have days when their motivation lags. Here are some suggestions to help you stick to your exercise regimen:

Make workouts enjoyable
- Choose an activity or sport that you like.
- Join a team sport or activity.
- Participate with a friend or family member.
- Vary exercise activities and routines.
- Vary exercise environments (e.g., walk, bike, or hike in areas you enjoy).
- Listen to music or audiobooks or watch a favorite television program while you exercise.

Sneak in workouts
- Take the stairs instead of elevators or escalators.
- Park far from store entrances and walk.
- Make several trips (e.g., loading and unloading the car).
- Walk or bike instead of driving short trips.
- Play, walk, bike, or hike with children or grandchildren.
- Walk or play with a pet.
- Work around the home (e.g., gardening and raking).

Exercises for the feet and lower legs

It is easy to incorporate some basic exercises into daily routines to help maintain the healthy function of the feet and lower legs. In fact, some of the exercises described below can be done just about anytime. They should, however, be combined with other activities to maintain total body strength, flexibility, balance, and cardiovascular fitness.

Sand walking—the perfect exercise

Earlier in the book, we discussed how unstable surfaces such as sand or excessively cushioned shoes can strain the feet and legs. However, when done safely, we can actually use the strain of sand to help build balance and endurance as part of a fitness routine. In fact, walking barefoot in loose sand is great way to exercise your feet. The natural, shifting surface of sand forces the feet, legs, and heart to work harder. You get strength training, flexibility, and aerobics all in one simple workout. What's more, the friction of the sand helps remove dry skin and calluses from the feet! Even a few minutes of sand walking as part of a normal workout routine can have tremendous benefits. If you don't live near a sandy beach, you can get some of the same benefits by walking barefoot on grass or similar soft surface. Short intervals of five to ten minutes each, as a part of a regular fitness routine, will give you the best results. Ideally, five to ten minutes of sand walking should be incorporated into a thirty- to sixty-minute walk once or twice a week. For those with better stamina, longer or more frequent sand walking intervals can be done.

Done regularly, sand walking will:

- strengthen your muscles.
- stretch your tendons and ligaments.
- elevate your heart rate (cardiovascular exercise).
- improve your balance.
- extend your range of motion.
- exfoliate the skin of your feet.

There are, of course, a few cautions for walking barefoot in sand or in grass. Make sure to walk in an area free of debris and inspect the bottoms of your feet afterward. Avoid sand that is uncomfortably hot, as it can burn the feet. Wearing flexible beach footwear offers protection while still allowing enough movement to exercise the feet and lower legs. Avoid walking barefoot outdoors if you suffer from numbness in your feet; but if you do go sand walking, wear protective footwear and inspect your feet frequently. Also avoid sand walking if you have an injury, arthritis, or history of falling.

Stretching the calf and Achilles tendon

Stretching should be a part of every fitness routine. It helps soothe sore muscles and maintain flexibility. It is not necessary to stretch aggressively. Slow, gentle movements, performed regularly, lengthen and strengthen muscles, tendons, and other soft tissues and help them maintain their elasticity. Stretching after a brief warm-up exercise, such as after walking or jogging in place for five minutes, is safer and more comfortable than stretching without warming up, especially if you are not very limber. Stretching should be done at least once a day and is most effective when combined with range-of-motion exercises, such as those described below.

Stretching the Achilles tendon

Stretching the Achilles tendon helps decrease calf pain, heel pain, and forefoot pain. The Achilles tendon is responsible for transmitting to the feet 80 percent of the step force generated by the legs. If the Achilles tendon is too tight, pressure is increased on the heel, the plantar fascia, the arch, and the ball of the foot.

Technically, you do not stretch your Achilles tendon but the muscles attached to the tendon. There are two stretches you can use to stretch these muscles. One involves leaning against a wall, counter, or similar vertical object; the other involves standing on stairs.

To stretch the Achilles tendon using the first exercise, face a wall or similar firm structure and place both hands against it, about shoulder height, with your elbows extended. Place one foot about twelve inches from the wall and extend the other leg behind you. The extended leg is the one that you will be stretching. With your extended foot flat on the ground, place your body weight on it, leaning slightly forward, until a stretching sensation is felt in the calf. Adjust the leg's distance from the wall and the weight you're

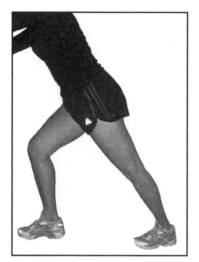

Calf stretch with knee straight.

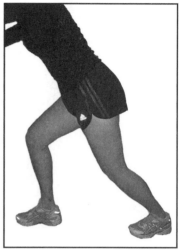

Calf stretch with knee bent.

placing on it until the stretch begins to feel slightly uncomfortable. For many people, this initial distance is about three feet. Those with greater flexibility will have to extend the leg farther from the wall to feel the stretch. Do not, however, stretch to the point of pain. Hold the stretch for thirty seconds with your leg straight and your knee locked. Then bend your knee and hold the stretch for another thirty seconds. When your knee is bent, the stretch should feel lower on the calf, closer to your heel, than when your knee is straight.

One calf may feel tighter than the other. This is normal and usually evens out with regular stretching and exercise. Sometimes relaxing and restretching helps relieve cramped or achy muscles. But, as I noted above, do not stretch to the point of pain. In fact, you should not even attempt to stretch an injured muscle or tendon unless you are under the care of a physician or physical therapist. Stretching a muscle or tendon too much or too often can actually damage the soft tissue, so immediately stop stretching if you feel pain.

Stretching your Achilles tendon on stairs may be easier for you, but it also can increase the risk of injury. More of your body weight will be pressing on your foot in this stretch, so perform it very cautiously until you are comfortable and confident doing it. For greater safety, perform this stretch on a staircase with a handrail.

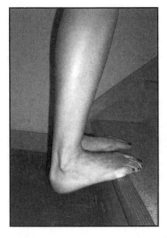 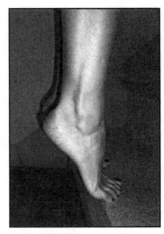

Calf stretch on stairs. Be careful to steady yourself by grasping the handrails firmly.

To begin, step up onto one of the stairs with both feet while facing upstairs and grasping the handrail for balance. Then slowly slide your feet back until your heels are hanging off the edge of the stair. Keeping your knees straight, slowly lower your heels until a gentle tension is felt in the calf. Hold this position for thirty seconds. Next, slightly bend your knees and gently lower your heels, stretching again for thirty seconds. This stretch can be done with both legs at the same time or one leg at a time, depending on what feels comfortable and stable to you.

An added bonus of this stretch is that the calf muscles can be strengthened with just a slight change to the stretching routine. The calf muscles stretch and lengthen as the heel is lowered and contract as the heel is raised, so incorporating ten heel raises after the stretch can strengthen the calf very effectively, while adding less than a minute to the routine.

Stretching the bottoms of the feet

Stretching the structures on the bottom of the feet can help alleviate arch strain, plantar fasciitis, and fatigued feet. This stretch can be done while sitting or standing. The toes and ball of one foot are placed against the base of a wall. Press the foot toward the floor until a gentle tension is felt on the bottom of the arch. A single stretch, held for fifteen to thirty seconds, is usually sufficient. Alternate feet to complete the stretch.

Stretching the foot can be done with or without the shoe on.

Range-of-motion exercises

The term *range of motion* refers to how fully a joint can freely move. As we age, our joints tend to lose their range of motion, and this can, in turn, place more stress on our soft tissues and bones. Arthritic conditions, tight muscles, and old injuries can further decrease range of motion. Exercise helps improve and maintain range of motion, including range of motion in joints affected by sprains, tendonitis, or general stiffness.

For the best results, range-of-motion exercises and stretching should be done in combination. Some people find that they are more comfortable stretching after they have done their range-of-motion exercises, while others prefer stretching first. Still others find that if they stretch, do range-of-motion exercises, and then stretch again, their flexibility is noticeably improved. Experiment with range-of-motion exercises and stretches until you find a sequence that works for you.

Preserving or increasing range of motion can be done by consciously moving the joints on a regular basis. The joints in the feet and lower legs that will benefit most from range-of-motion exercises are the ankle joint, the subtalar joint, and the midtarsal joint. Fortunately they can all be moved with one easy exercise. This exercise not only moves the foot and ankle through its entire range of motion but also helps strengthen the muscles that move the foot and lower leg.

The exercise is done with one foot at a time while seated. Raise one foot off the ground about three to six inches. Next, write the alphabet in the air with the toes, making sure to move the foot at the ankle and exaggerate the shape of the letters. Most of the movement should occur from the ankle and down. Some movements or letters may be more difficult than others. Remember these and repeat them. Switch feet and repeat. This exercise can be done once daily for range-of-motion maintenance or up to three times daily if recovering from a foot or ankle injury.

Another exercise can be done in conjunction with this range-of-motion exercise (or whenever seated). This exercise will maintain or increase the flexibility and range of motion of the forefoot, especially the big toe joint. To perform this exercise, first take off your shoes. Place both feet flat on the floor, then raise your heels off the ground while keeping your forefoot and toes on the floor. This exercise forces the toe joints at the ball of the feet to bend while also stretching the soft structures of the arch and heel. Most people can do this exercise quite easily. Repeat thirty to fifty times or for sixty seconds to maintain range of motion and flexibility of the forefoot and arch. I especially recommend this exercise for those prone to plantar fasciitis.

Strengthening exercises

There are many benefits to strengthening the muscles of the feet and lower legs. Stronger muscles mean that you're less likely to fall, suffer a stress fracture, or develop a condition like plantar fasciitis. As I've noted previously, wearing shoes can cause the muscles of the feet to atrophy over time, and since most of us wear shoes most of the time, just about everyone benefits from strength training for the feet and legs.

You can strengthen your calf muscles by doing calf raises while standing on a stair or while seated. Calf raises are done exactly as their name suggests: you simply raise your heels from the ground, contracting the large muscle group that makes up the calf. Some people combine the calf stair-stretch exercises described earlier with the calf strengthening exercise to save time. The calf is stretched when the heel is lowered, and the calf is strengthened when the heel is raised.

The muscles on the bottom of the feet can be difficult to isolate, but there are three simple exercises you can do to strengthen them. These exercises are especially beneficial if you have plantar fasciitis. The first two exercises are done sitting down and barefoot. The third can be done barefoot or in shoes, at any time, standing or sitting.

For the first exercise, lay a towel down at your bare feet. Grasp the towel with your toes and slowly draw the towel toward the heels. Repeat this movement five to ten times for each foot. As the exercise becomes easier for you, increase the number of repetitions you are doing or stack weights on the towel for extra resistance.

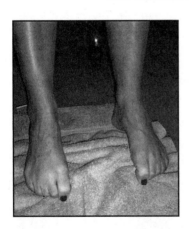

Curling your toes as you draw a towel toward you will strengthen your arch muscles.

For the second exercise, pick up marbles with your bare toes and drop them into a bucket one by one while seated. Do this for five to ten minutes once a day or every other day.

The final exercise can be done without removing your shoes. Curl your toes and raise the arch of your foot by pressing your toes into the bottoms of your shoes. Hold this position for two seconds, relax, then repeat ten to twenty times for each foot. You should feel some fatigue in your arch muscles when finished.

Balance exercises

Balance can be improved by "exercising" the small nerves called proprioceptors that help the feet and ankles sense the ground and the body's position in space. Balancing on one foot is a great way to exercise the proprioceptors and muscles around the ankle. To be safe, you should balance barefoot on a firm and level surface within a door frame or next to a chair or counter to prevent yourself from falling if you should lose your balance. Wearing shoes or standing on a carpet can make it more difficult for your body to sense the surface properly. If foot pain prevents you from exercising barefoot, use a thin rug or wear supportive footwear.

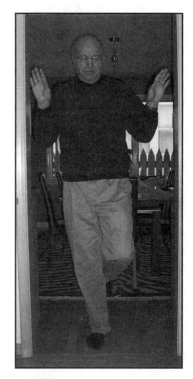

Begin the exercise by standing on one leg for as long as you can—your goal being to stand for one full minute. Repeat with your other leg. Do the exercise daily until you can easily balance for one minute. Then, gradually increase the balancing time on each leg from one to four minutes, in increments of a minute at a time. It may take a few weeks to build up to four minutes, so be patient.

Once you can balance comfortably for four minutes at a time on each foot, try to work your way from one minute to four minutes again, but this time with your eyes closed. When you remove the visual feedback your open eyes provide, your

Balancing on one leg is safer if you stand in a doorway with your hands ready to brace yourself should you lose your balance.

Risk Factors for Falling

Personal Factors	Environmental Factors
alcohol consumption arthritis balance disorder cardiac disease dementia hypertension impaired health muscle weakness peripheral neuropathy side effect of medication unwillingness to use a walker or cane vascular disease visual impairment	poor walking surface (icy, wet, steep, uneven, unstable, etc.) challenging obstacles poor footwear bad lighting

proprioceptors must work much harder. Be careful, though. Open your eyes at the first sensation of falling.

To exercise your proprioceptors, you might also experiment with Tai Chi Ch'uan. This Asian form of exercise has been shown to improve balance and reduce the risk of falling.[27] Its precise, graceful movements strengthen, stretch, and relax the body. Many health clubs or recreation centers offer Tai Chi classes.

Preventing falls

According to the American Geriatrics Society, as many as 40 percent of those 65 and older who are in good health fall each year.[28] This risk of falling increases with age. Most falls result in only minor injuries, such as cuts or bruises, but more serious falls can cause fractures or head injuries. The psychological harm, however, can be more devastating than the physical injury, leading to loss of confidence and, as a result, decreased activity.

Most falls not related to playing sports occur while walking or going down stairs. Nearly half are caused by slipping or tripping. Many falls are caused by a combination of contributing factors that increase the likelihood of slipping or tripping. A number of these contributing factors are age related, including slowing reflexes, deteriorating balance, failing vision, increasing joint pain, declining muscle strength, and decreasing flexibility. You can minimize the effects of these age-related factors and reduce your risk of falling by becoming more fit, wearing better footwear, using walking aids, and addressing both the personal and environmental factors that contribute to falling.

Sometimes problems with balance or falling can signal a serious medical condition, such as peripheral neuropathy, dementia, a nutritional or circulation disorder, an aneurysm, a brain tumor, or an adverse drug reaction. See a physician if you are experiencing persistent balance or falling problems.

If you want to develop a comprehensive plan for preventing falls, consider all the following:

- physical changes to the home (installing hand rails and grab bars, rearranging furniture, removing clutter, improving lighting, and converting to nonslip flooring)
- medication management (adjusting dosages, avoiding medications that are known to cause dizziness, being alert to possible drug interactions)
- assistive devices (cane, walker)
- exercise (strength training, flexibility)
- footwear

For the purposes of this section, I will focus on the relationship between footwear and falling. Most falls occur while wearing footwear simply because we almost always wear shoes when we are up and about. But footwear is a contributing factor in many falls.

Footwear and falls

Several studies have found that footwear is a significant factor in up to half of all falls in older patients. A study done at Stanford University, for example, found that wearing high-heeled shoes not only increased the risk of falling but also of breaking a bone as a result of the fall.[29] The following problems with footwear all contribute to the risk of falling:

- poor fit
- unsecured heel straps or untied laces
- heels that are too high
- soft shoes
- excessively worn shoes
- slippery soles
- heavy shoes

Poorly fitting shoes that are too large can slip and slide on the foot or catch at the toe when walking. Shoes that are too tight constrict the feet and cause pain, both of which decrease stability. Open-heeled shoes are easy to slip onto the feet and work well for people who have difficulty bending or tying laces, but they are also more likely to cause falls than shoes that are more secure. Soft shoes compress each step, impairing balance and increasing step impact.[30] Old, worn-out shoes tend to be too loose. Their stretched uppers fail to hold feet securely, so the feet slip from side to side. Old shoes often have less traction and uneven outsoles. Slippery and worn soles, especially in certain weather conditions, are one of the most common footwear problems. For those who have some leg weakness or fatigue easily, heavier shoes can cause the feet to "drag," which may lead to tripping.

Shoes and traction

Choose shoes that offer traction that is appropriate for the surface you are walking on, weather conditions, and your walking gait. In general, shoes with more surface area on the soles provide better traction—and, therefore, are more likely to prevent falls—than shoes with less surface area. A larger surface area also provides more stability under the feet. Patterned, textured, and treaded soles and soles made of rubber and other nonslip materials provide better traction than smooth leather soles.

Consider the weather conditions when you go to the closet to select the shoes you're going to wear. When it's wet and slick outside, or snowy and icy, your risk of falling increases substantially. Choose shoes with textured rubber outsoles for these conditions. Traction can be also enhanced by wearing rubber overshoes (galoshes) or shoe devices such as Yaktrax, a slip-on rubber-and-wire traction device that can be easily attached to provide safer footing.

While it may seem that the more traction you have, the better, this is not always the case. Sometimes, too much traction can create a tripping hazard. Parkinson's and other medical conditions can force people to shuffle their feet. If they are wearing shoes with excessive traction, their feet can catch and they can trip and fall.

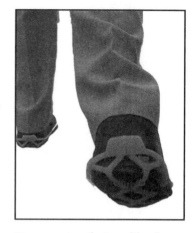

Foot traction devices, like the one above by Yaktrax, can lower the risk of falling in slippery conditions. The device attaches to the bottom of the shoe.

To stay active, you need to keep your feet healthy. The simple stretching, strengthening, and balancing exercises in this chapter should be a part of your regular exercise program, especially if you are prone to foot injuries or problems. And since the risk of falls increases as we age, the link between healthy feet and good balance becomes even more important over time. Take good care of your feet and you'll have a firm foundation for years of happy, healthy living.

Footcare Products and Resources

The foot health industry is booming, and with this boom comes an ever-growing variety of footcare products. The products described in this chapter and elsewhere in the book are some of the more useful ones available. Most can be purchased in pharmacies, shoe stores, and footcare centers; through mail-order catalogs; or over the Internet. An index of footcare-related Internet sites is included at the end of this chapter.

Foot spas and whirlpool baths

A number of foot spas are commercially available, ranging in price from $20 to over $100. The spas offer such features as vibrating massagers, water jets, infrared heat, and remote controls. While soaking the feet is rarely the primary treatment of choice for most sources of foot pain or injury, foot spas do offer benefits for tired, achy feet and some skin conditions. The warm water and massaging action can also decrease pain from arthritis and circulation disorders.

Soaking the feet can also soften the skin and nails. In fact, many people have found that soaking the feet for fifteen to thirty minutes before caring for calluses or trimming the toenails makes the task much easier. Keep in mind that soaking the skin can actually contribute to drier skin, so applying a lotion to the feet after soaking

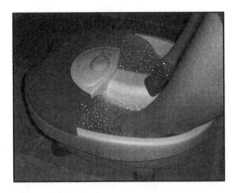

Soaking helps soothe the feet and makes skin and nail care easier.

can help preserve the natural moisture level of the skin.

Do not use a foot spa if you have an open sore on your foot. And you should not share a foot spa with others due to the risk of contamination and infection. Injured or swollen feet should not be soaked in warm or hot water as this can increase swelling and inflammation. Also, if you have neuropathy, be very careful about immersing your feet in hot water.

Foot massagers

Tired, aching feet can be rejuvenated with massage. Some foot injuries, such as plantar fasciitis, can also benefit from gentle rubbing. Foot massagers come in all shapes and sizes, from low tech to high tech. Simple wooden rollers, rubber knobs, or even tennis balls can be used to gently massage the bottoms of the feet while sitting. More expensive foot massagers may use vibration, heat, motorized rollers, or "acupressure" to soothe the feet.

The best foot massagers can be used when sitting. This allows you to control some of the pressure exerted against your feet. Massaging slippers or insoles are promoted by some manufactures for their health benefits, but because they are used when standing or walking, the pressure on the feet may be too great. Also, massaging slippers or insoles are intended only for short-term use. If you wear them too long, you may actually experience more discomfort than relief.

Cushioned socks

Padded stockings are becoming increasingly common. They can be useful for those who prefer not to wear shoes in the house or who are vulnerable to pressure-related pain on the bottoms of their feet. Some padded stockings have an extra thick layer of fabric; others incorporate a silicone pad in the forefoot and heel. Studies have shown that there is less pressure on the feet when wearing padded socks versus regular socks.

Sock-donning aid

As we age, putting on socks and stockings can become more and more difficult. Back pain, obesity, arthritis, and swelling can all conspire to make it harder for you to reach your feet. Compression stockings can be especially difficult to put on. Fortunately, there is a simple device that can help. A sock-donning aid is a plastic U-shaped tube with a rope handle attached. This device can make the chore of putting on socks and stockings much easier. The socks are slipped over the tube, and the handle is used to pull the socks up over the toes and ankles. The tube then slides off the back of the feet, and the socks can be pulled up to the calf.

Footbathing aids

To decrease the risk of athlete's foot, dry skin, and fungal toenails, you need to wash your feet regularly. However, as noted above, our ability to reach our feet can become constrained as we age. A simple, soft foot-scrubbing device can be placed on the floor of the tub or shower. After applying soap, gently rub your feet against the rubbery foot scrubber and then rinse.

Long-handled lotion applicators

Applying lotion to the feet is much easier if you use a lotion applicator. The applicator cannot rub the lotion into the skin quite as well as your own hands, but it does get lotion to places that you otherwise could not reach. This device is especially useful for those who do not have a family member or caregiver who can assist them.

Internet foot health resources and products

You may find the following Web sites helpful as you search for information about foot conditions, footwear, and foot health products. The list is by no means exhaustive, and inclusion on the list does not signify an endorsement of the information, products, or services offered. A more up-to-date list can be found at www.greatfeetforlife.com.

Foot health information

American Academy of Podiatric Sports Medicine: www.aapsm.org

American Association of Retired Persons: www.aarp.org

American College of Foot and Ankle Surgeons: www.acfas.org

American Diabetes Association: www.diabetes.org

American Orthopaedic Foot and Ankle Society: www.aofas.org

American Podiatric Medical Association: www.apma.org

Centers for Disease Control and Prevention: www.cdc.gov

Epodiatry.com

Foot Health Care: www.foothealthcare.com

Foot Health Foundation of America: www.foothealthfdn.org

Foot Health Network: www.foot.com

Great Feet for Life: www.greatfeetforlife.com

Health and Age: www.healthandage.com

National Institute of Arthritis and Musculoskeletal and Skin
      Diseases: www.niams.nih.gov

National Institutes of Health: www.nih.gov

National Institute on Aging: www.grc.nia.nih.gov

Pedorthic Footwear Association: www.pedorthics.org

Savvy Senior: www.savvysenior.org

WebMD: www.webmd.com

Footcare products

Activeforever.com

Dr. Scholls: www.drscholls.com

Elderdepot.com

Footexpress.com
Footsmart.com
Hapad.com
Healthyfeetstore.com
Myfootshop.com
Shoefootandbody.com
Thebonestore.com
Yaktrax: www.yaktrax.com

Footwear retailers

Eneslow Foot Comfort Center: www.eneslow.com
Foot Solutions: www.footsolutions.com
Footwear etc.: www.footwearetc.com
Payless Shoe Source: www.payless.com
Schuler Shoes: www.schulershoes.com
Shoes-n-Feet: www.shoesnfeet.com
The Walking Company: www.thewalkingcompany.com
Tradehome Shoes: www.tradehome.com

Custom footwear

Otabo: www.otabo.com

Footwear manufacturers

Adidas: www.adidas.com
Aetrex: www.aetrex.com
Airwalk: www.airwalk.com
Aravon: www.aravonshoes.com
Asics: www.asicsamerica.com
Beautifeel: www.beautifeel.com
Birkenstock: www.birkenstock.com
Born: www.bornshoes.com
Brooks: www.brooksrunning.com
Chaco: www.chacousa.com

Clark's: www.clarks.co.uk
Cole Haan: www.colehaan.com
Crocs: www.crocsrx.com
Dansko: www.dansko.com
Dexter: www.dextershoe.com
Dockers: www.dockersshoes.com
Drew: www.drewshoe.com
Earth Shoes: www.earth.us
Ecco: www.ecco.com
Etonic: www.etonic.com
Finn Comfort: www.finncomfort.de
Haflinger: www.haflinger.com
Keen: www.keenfootwear.com
MBT: www.mbt-info.com
Mephisto: www.mephisto,com
Merrell: www.merrellboot.com
Mizuno: www.mizunousa.com
Munro: www.munroshoe.com
Naot: www.naot.com
New Balance: www.newbalance.com
Nike: www.nike.com
P.W. Minor: www.pwminor.com
Puma: www.puma.com
Red Wing: www.redwing.com
Reebok: www.reebok.com
Rockport: www.rockport.com
San Antonio Shoes (SAS): www.sasshoes.com
Saucony: www.saucony.com
Taryn Rose, M.D.: www.tarynrose.com
Teva: www.teva.com
Think!: www.thinkshoes.com
Ugg: www.uggaustralia.com
Wolky: www.wolky.com

Insole manufacturers

Insolia: www.insolia.com
Power*step*: www.powersteps.com
Sof Sole: www.sofsole.com
Spenco: www.spenco.com
Superfeet: www.superfeet.com
Tacco: www.tacco.de

Socks and compression stockings

Goldtoe: www.goldtoebrands.com
Jobst compression stockings: www.jobst-usa.com
Smartwool: www.smartwool.com
Wigwam: www.wigwam.com

Notes

1. Lazaro, P, et al., "Dermatologic diseases and podiatric disorders in the feet of elderly populations: a descriptive study," *Journal of the European Academy of Dermatology and Venereology*, 17 (3): 274, 2003 Nov.
2. Helfand, AE, "Geriatric primary podiatric medicine," *Clinics in Podiatric Medicine and Surgery*, 20 (3): 583-591, 2003.
3. Ounpoo, S, Gage, JR, Davis, RB, "Three-dimensional lower extremity joint kinematics in normal pediatric gait," *Journal of Pediatric Orthopaedics*, 11 (3): 341–349, 1991.
4. Lazaro, P, et al., "Dermatologic diseases and podiatric disorders."
5. Benvenuti, F, et al., "Foot pain and disability in older persons: an epidemiologic survey," *Journal of the American Geriatrics Society*, 43 (5): 479–484, 1995 May.
6. Helfand, AE, "Foot pain in later life: some psychosocial correlates," *Clinics in Podiatric Medicine and Surgery*, 20 (3): 395–406, 2003.
7. Focht, DR, Spicer, C, Fairchok, MP, "The efficacy of duct tape vs. cryotherapy in the treatment of verruca vulgaris," *Archives of Pediatric and Adolescent Medicine*, 156 (10): 971–974, 2002 Oct.
8. Warshaw, EM, St. Clair, KR, "Prevention of onychomycosis reinfection for patients with complete cure of all ten toenails: results of a double-blind, placebo-controlled pilot study of prophylactic miconazole powder 2%," *Journal of the American Academy of Dermatology*, 53 (4): 717–720, 2005 Oct.

9. Warshaw, EM, "Prevention of reinfection in patients successfully treated for toenail onychomycosis: results of a double-blind, randomized, placebo-controlled trial," *Journal of the American Academy of Dermatology*, 50 (3): 102, 2004.

10. *American Heart Association Disease and Stroke Statistics 2005 Update*, American Heart Association, 1–61.

11. Priplata, AA, Niemi, JB, Harry, JD, Lipsitz, LA, Collins, JJ, "Vibrating insoles and balance control in elderly people," *Lancet*, 362 (9390): 1123-1124, 2003 Oct.

12. Hoffman, P, "Conclusions drawn from a comparative study of the feet of barefooted and shoe-wearing peoples," *Journal of Bone and Joint Surgery*, 3: 105–136, 1905.

13. Schulman, S, "Survey in China and India of feet that have never worn shoes," *Journal of the National Association of Chiropodists*, 49: 26–30, 1949.

14. Chantelau, E, Gede, A, "Foot dimensions of elderly people with and without diabetes mellitus: a data basis for shoe design," *Gerontology*, 48 (4): 241–244, 2002.

15. Robbins, SE, et al., "Aging in relation to optimization of footwear in older men," *Journal of the American Geriatrics Society*, 45 (1): 61–67, 1997.

16. Miller, JE, Nigg, BM, Liu, W, Stefanyshyn, DJ, Nurse, MA, "Influence of foot, leg and shoe characteristics on subjective comfort," *Foot and Ankle International*, 21 (9): 759–767, 2000 Sept.

17. Frey, C, Thompson, F, et al., "American Orthopedic Foot and Ankle Society's Women's Shoe Survey," *Foot & Ankle*, 14 (2): 78–81, 1993 Feb.

18. Menz, HB, Morris, ME, "Footwear characteristics and foot problems in older people," *Gerontology*, 51 (5): 346–351, 2005 Sept.

19. Lord, SR, Bashford, GM, "Shoe characteristics and balance in older women," *Journal of the American Geriatric Society*, 44 (4): 429–433, 1996 Apr.

20. Chantelau E, Gede A, "Foot dimensions of elderly people."

21. Newbalance.com, August 8, 2006.

22. Nigg, B, Hintzen, S, Ferber, R, "Effect of an unstable shoe construction on lower extremity gait characteristics," *Clinical Biomechanics*, 21 (1): 82–88, 2006.

23. Finlay O, "Replacing elderly patient's ill-fitting shoes has benefits for both patients and health services," *Health Service Journal*, 31, February 8, 1996.

24. *The Heidelberg Guidelines for Promoting Physical Activity Among Older Persons*, World Health Organization, 1996.

25. Adab, P, Macfarlane, DJ, "Exercise and health—new imperatives for public health policy in Hong Kong," *Hong Kong Medical Journal*, 4 (4): 389–393, 1998.

26. U.S. Department of Health and Human Services, *Physical Activity and Health: A Report of the Surgeon General*, U.S. Department of Health and Human Services, Centers for Disease Control and Prevention, National Center for Chronic Disease Prevention and Health Promotion, 1996.

27. Wolf, SL, Barnhart, HX, Kutner, NG, McNeely, E, Coogler, C, Xu, T, "Reducing frailty and falls in older persons: an investigation of Tai Chi and computerized balance training," *Journal of the American Geriatric Society*, 44 (5): 489–97, 1996 May.

28. American Geriatrics Society, British Geriatrics Society and American Academy of Orthopaedic Surgeons Panel on Falls Prevention, "Guidelines for the prevention of falls in older persons," *Journal of the American Geriatrics Society*, 49: 664–672, 2001.

29. Keegan, T, et al., "Characteristics of fallers who fracture at the foot, distal forearm, proximal humerus, pelvis, and shaft of the tibia/fibula compared to fallers who do not fracture," *American Journal of Epidemiology*, 159 (2): 192–203, 2004.

30. Robbins, SE, Gouw, GJ, McClaran, J, "Shoe sole hardness and thickness influence balance in older men," *Journal of the American Geriatrics Society*, 40 (11): 1089–1094, 1992 Nov.

Glossary

accessory bone: extra bone(s) usually small and round, sometimes called ossicle

Achilles tendon: tendon that attaches to the back of the heel

additional-depth shoes: shoes with added depth to the toe box

anti-inflammatory medication: oral medication, such as ibuprofen and naproxen, that controls pain and inflammation; common brand names include Motrin and Aleve

artery: a blood vessel that carries blood away from the heart

athlete's foot: fungal infection affecting the skin of the feet; also called tinea pedis

atrophy: deterioration or shrinking of a soft-tissue structure such as muscle

big toe: the largest toe; also called the great toe or hallux

bone spur: a prominence of bone resulting from soft-tissue stress or injury

bony prominence: a bone or portion of bone that protrudes

bunion: an enlargement of the joint at the base of the big toe

bunionette: an enlargement of the joint at the base of the fifth toe

calcaneus: the heel bone

callus: thick layer of skin resulting from excessive pressure or friction

capsule: the soft tissue structures that envelope a joint

capsulitis: inflammation of the joint capsule

contusion: bruise

corn: *See* callus.

cuboid bone: square bone located in the midfoot

cuneiform bones: three bones (medial, middle, and lateral) located in the midfoot

erythema: redness and warmth to skin, usually accompanies inflammation or infection

exfoliating agent: an ingredient such as uric acid or lactic acid that is added to lotions or creams to gently dissolve dry skin

fibula: one of two long bones located between the knee and ankle

fifth toe: the smallest toe

first toe: the biggest toe

flat feet: feet with arches that collapse excessively under the weight of the body, potentially causing instability and pain

foot bed: an over-the-counter support that is placed in the shoe, also called an insole

fourth toe: the toe next to the smallest (or fifth) toe

fracture: a break or crack, usually used when referring to injured bone

fungal infection: *See* tinea pedis; athlete's foot; onychomycosis.

fungal nail: *See* onychomycosis.

ganglion: a benign fluid-filled cyst

granuloma: an inflamed, enlarged capillary bed that protrudes through the skin, also called a pyogenic granuloma

great toe: the largest toe; also called the big toe or hallux

hallux: the largest toe; also called the big toe or great toe

hallux limitus/rigidus: arthritis of the joint at the base of the big toe

heel spur: a prominence of bone usually on the bottom of the heel, commonly associated with plantar fasciitis

heel spur syndrome: *See* plantar fasciitis.

hyperhydrosis: a condition where the skin is moist due to excessive perspiration

incurvated nail: a nail that bends or curves at the corners; often precedes an ingrown nail

infection: invasion of the body by bacteria, fungi, or viruses

inflammation: the body's initial response to injury or infection, marked by redness, warmth, swelling, and pain

ingrown nail: a nail that has penetrated the skin, sometimes causing infection

insole: an over-the-counter foot bed placed in shoes to cushion or support the feet

last: the form that the shoe is wrapped around during the manufacture process; also, the shape of the shoe, from straight to semi-straight to semi-curved to curved

lateral: away from the midline or toward the side (for example, the little toe is lateral to the big toe)

ligament: a soft-tissue structure that attaches one bone to another bone

maceration: pale, sloughing, weakened skin, usually found between the toes due to excessive moisture or infection. *See also* hyperhydrosis.

malleolus: the ankle bone

medial: toward the midline (for example, the big toe is medial to the little toe)

metatarsal: the longest bones of the feet, the five metatarsals correspond with the five digits

nail bed: the skin under the toenail

nail border: the edge of the toenail

navicular: the boat-shaped bone in the midfoot

onychomycosis: an infection of the toenail caused by fungus, usually painless but causing discoloration, thickening, and a brittle texture of the nail

orthotics: foot support devices that are placed in the shoe, made from a cast of the foot

ossicle: an extra bone, usually small and round; also called the accessory bone

overpronation: a foot that pronates (i.e., flexes to absorb the weight of the body) excessively, potentially causing instability and pain. *See also* pronation.

peroneal tendon: one of three tendons on the lateral aspect of the lower leg and ankle

plantar fascia: a band of thick connective tissue that supports that arch of the foot

plantar fasciitis: inflammation of the plantar fascia

plantar fat pad: the layer of fat on the bottom of the foot that helps absorb step impact

porokeratosis: a type of callus on the bottom of the foot that has a hard center

posterior tibial tendon: a large muscle-tendon unit originating to the back of the calf and attaching to the bottom of the foot's arch

pronation: a complex movement of the joints of the foot and ankle that occurs as the heel strikes the ground when walking or running; allows the foot to absorb impact and adapt to the walking or running surface; the collapse of the arch is one component of pronation

Raynaud's disease/phenomenon: a spastic disorder of the small blood vessels in the fingers and toes triggered by cold

second toe: the toe next to the big toe

sesamoid bones: small, seed-like bones located in pairs under the first metatarsal phalangeal joint

spur: *See* bone spur *or* heel spur.

stress fracture: a break in a bone that is not caused by trauma

stress reaction: a condition of the bone that precedes a stress fracture

supination: a complex movement of the foot and ankle joints that occurs as weight is transferred to the forefoot during walking or running; the arch rises and the foot locks in order to provide a firm foundation to propel the leg forward

tendon: a soft-tissue structure that attaches muscle to bone

third toe: the middle toe

tibia: one of two long bones of the lower leg, located between the knee and ankle

tinea pedis: fungal infection of the skin of the feet, also called athlete's foot

ulcer: an open sore

varicose veins: veins that have enlarged and become visible through the skin

vein: a blood vessel that carries blood to the heart

venous stasis: pooling of blood in the lower legs caused by sluggish flow in the veins

venous stasis ulceration: a breakdown of the skin on the lower legs caused by the chronic swelling associated with venous stasis

Index

A

accessory bone (ossicle), 192, 196

acetaminophen, 70

Achilles tendon, 66, 68, 74, 164, 170–172, 193; and Haglund's bumps, 69, 147; calcification of (posterior heel spurs), 68–69; stretching, 66, 170–171; inflammation of (Achilles tendonitis), 68, 147, 164

Achilles tendonitis, 68, 147, 164

additional-depth shoes, 19, 36, 86, 120–121, 124

allergic reaction, 14, 19, 20, 21–22, 24

allergy, 17. *See also* allergic reaction

alpha hydroxyl acid lotion, 15

American Diabetes Association, 184

American Orthopaedic Foot and Ankle Society, 184

American Podiatric Medical Association, 1, 109, 184

ankle, 10, 61, 122, 126, 128, 135, 152, 172, 173, 194, 196, 197; and Achilles tendonitis, 68; and balance, 175; and collar height, 135; and fallen arches (PTTD), 71-72; and peripheral neuropathy, 103; and shoe inserts, 154; and socks, 148, 183; and tarsal tunnel syndrome, 106; arthritis in, 71, 73; bone (malleolus), 196; brace, 147; collapsing, 126;

conditions and injuries, 60,62, 63, 124; edema (swelling) in, 93, 96, 148; joint, 61, 173; pain, 147; orthotic, 106; skin changes in, 94; sprain, 6, 7, 57, 58, 70–71, 106, 142; support, 124, 127, 154

antibacterial insoles, 158

antifungal medication, 13, 16, 18, 23, 54, 56; oral, 48, 54, 56; powder, 17, 18; topical, 13, 48, 51, 54

anti-inflammatory medication, 64, 67, 68, 69, 70, 73, 75, 79, 80, 81, 82, 98, 99, 105, 106, 193

aperture pad, 35, 161

arch, 2, 4, 60, 62, 63, 123, 141, 170; and arthritis, 146; and exercise, 67; and plantar fasciitis, 64, 147; blisters on (athlete's foot), 18, 19; collapsing, 64, 72, 74, 88, 106, 154, 157, 160, 194, 196; fallen (PTTD), 6, 71–73, 145; flattening of, 6, 74; height of, 112; high, 6, 7, 8, 59, 122; low or flat, 7, 8, 59, 74, 122, 145, 194; normal or neutral, 7, 8, 122; padding, 33, 35, 36, 122, 160; pain in, 62, 74, 75, 106, 154, 158, 160; stretching, 172, 174, 175; support (insoles and orthotics), 33, 63, 64, 65, 68, 72, 73, 74, 78, 79, 92, 106, 112, 122, 131, 144, 148, 151, 152, 153, 157, 158, 159, 160–161, 163.